Expecting

Well

A Comprehensive Guide to a Healthy Pregnancy

By

Njenga Watathi

KDP ISBN: 9798393291907
Imprint: Independently published

Abstract

This book offers a detailed and informative guide for expectant mothers to have a healthy and happy pregnancy. The book covers a wide range of topics, including nutrition, exercise, common pregnancy symptoms, prenatal testing, and more. It also includes advice on managing stress, and emotions during pregnancy, as well as preparing for childbirth and the postpartum period. The author draws on the latest research in the field of obstetrics and gynecology to provide evidence-based advice and practical tips for a healthy pregnancy. The book is written in a clear and concise language, making it accessible to readers with varying levels of medical knowledge. With the help of this book, expectant mothers can make informed decisions about their health and the health of their baby. It provides them with the tools to create a personalized pregnancy plan that fits their individual needs and preferences. The book also emphasizes the importance of self-care during pregnancy, encouraging mothers to take care of their physical and emotional health. It is a comprehensive resource that empowers women to have a positive and healthy pregnancy experience. Therefore, this book is an essential read for any expectant mother who wants to ensure a healthy and happy pregnancy. It is a valuable resource for healthcare professionals, educators, and anyone else interested in promoting maternal and fetal health.

Table of Contents

1. How to Maintain a Healthy Diet during Pregnancy

1.1. Introduction

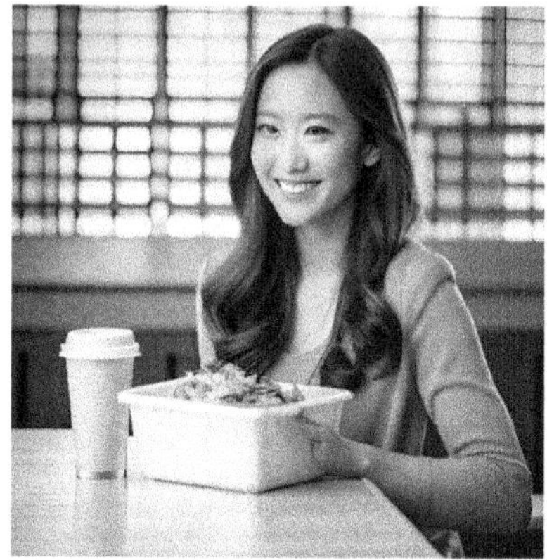

Pregnancy is a unique and life-changing experience for every woman. It is essential to maintain a healthy and balanced diet during this time to ensure the health and well-being of both the mother and the developing baby. This chapter will discuss some practical tips and tricks to help expectant mothers maintain a healthy diet during pregnancy.

1.2. Strategies for Maintaining a Healthy Diet

1. Eat a balanced diet

A balanced diet is essential for a healthy pregnancy. A balanced diet consists of a variety of foods that provide essential nutrients, including protein, carbohydrates, vitamins, and minerals. Some examples of nutrient-dense foods include fruits, vegetables, whole grains, lean protein, and dairy products. Pregnant women should aim to consume a variety of nutrient-dense foods to meet their daily nutritional needs.

Real-life example: Sarah, a pregnant mother, starts her day with a balanced breakfast consisting of whole-grain toast, scrambled eggs, and fruit. For lunch, she has a salad with grilled chicken, vegetables, and whole-grain bread. She snacks on fruit, nuts, or yogurt between meals. For dinner, she has grilled salmon, steamed vegetables, and quinoa. Sarah ensures that she consumes a variety of nutrient-dense foods throughout the day to meet her daily nutritional needs.

2. Consume enough calories

During pregnancy, the body requires extra calories to support the growth and development of the fetus. Pregnant women should aim to consume an additional 300-500 calories per day, depending on their pre-pregnancy weight and activity level. However, it is essential to note that not all calories are created equal, and pregnant women should aim to consume nutrient-dense calories.

Real-life example: Maria, a pregnant mother, is physically active and has a pre-pregnancy weight in the healthy range. She aims to consume an additional 300 calories per day, which equates to a small snack, such as an apple with almond butter or a small bowl of whole-grain cereal with milk.

3. Stay hydrated

Staying hydrated during pregnancy is essential for the health of the mother and the developing baby. Pregnant women should aim to consume at least 8-10 glasses of water per day. In addition to water, pregnant women can also consume other hydrating fluids, such as herbal tea, coconut water, or fresh fruit juice. However, it is important to limit the intake of caffeinated beverages, such as coffee and tea.

Real-life example: Lisa, a pregnant mother, carries a water bottle with her wherever she goes to ensure that she stays hydrated throughout the day. She also enjoys herbal tea and occasionally drinks fresh fruit juice as a hydrating alternative.

4. Limit processed and junk food

Processed and junk food is high in calories and low in nutrients. Consuming too much processed and junk food during pregnancy can lead to excessive weight gain, nutrient deficiencies, and an increased risk of gestational diabetes. Pregnant women should limit their intake of processed and junk food and opt for nutrient-dense foods instead.

Real-life example: Rachel, a pregnant mother, enjoys the occasional treat but makes an effort to limit her intake of processed and junk food. Instead, she opts for nutrient-dense snacks, such as fruit, vegetables with hummus, or Greek yogurt with berries.

5. Choose healthy fats

Healthy fats are an essential component of a healthy diet and are particularly important during pregnancy. Healthy fats, such as omega-3 fatty acids, are important for the development of the fetal brain and nervous system. Pregnant women should aim to consume healthy fats from sources such as oily fish, nuts, seeds, and avocados. Fats are an essential nutrient during pregnancy as they play a vital role in the development of the fetus's brain and nervous system. However, not all fats are created equal. Pregnant women should aim to consume healthy fats, such as monounsaturated and polyunsaturated fats, while avoiding unhealthy fats, such as trans fats. Good sources of healthy fats include olive oil, avocado, nuts, seeds, and fatty fish. Pregnant women should limit their intake of saturated fats, which are found in fatty meats and full-fat dairy products, as well as trans fats, which are found in processed and fried foods.

Real-life example: Lisa, a pregnant mother, chooses healthy fats by cooking with olive oil, snacking on nuts and seeds, and eating fatty fish like salmon once a week. She avoids processed and fried foods that contain trans fats.

6. Get enough protein

Protein is essential for the growth and development of the fetus and the placenta. Pregnant women should aim to consume at least 70-100 grams of protein per day, depending on their pre-pregnancy weight and activity level (American College of Obstetricians and Gynecologists. (2021). Nutrition during pregnancy). Good sources of protein include lean meat, fish, eggs, beans, lentils, and tofu.

Real-life example: Emily, a pregnant mother, makes an effort to consume protein-rich foods with every meal. For breakfast, she enjoys a smoothie made with Greek yogurt and fruit. For lunch, she has a salad with chicken, beans, and seeds. For dinner, she has grilled fish or tofu with vegetables.

7. Take prenatal vitamins

Prenatal vitamins are an essential component of a healthy pregnancy diet. Prenatal vitamins contain essential nutrients, such as folic acid, iron, calcium, and vitamin D that are necessary for the growth and development of the fetus. Pregnant women should take prenatal vitamins as directed by their healthcare provider.

Real-life example: Julia, a pregnant mother, takes a prenatal vitamin every day to ensure that she is getting all the essential nutrients she needs for a healthy pregnancy.

8. Avoid alcohol, smoking, and drugs

Alcohol, smoking, and drugs can have harmful effects on the developing fetus. Pregnant women should avoid alcohol, smoking, and drugs during pregnancy to reduce the risk of fetal alcohol syndrome, low birth weight, and other complications.

Real-life example: Sarah, a pregnant mother, quit smoking and drinking alcohol as soon as she found out she was pregnant. She also avoids exposure to secondhand smoke and drugs.

1.3. Conclusion

Maintaining a healthy diet during pregnancy is essential for the health and well-being of both the mother and the developing baby. Pregnant women should aim to eat a balanced diet, consume enough calories, stay hydrated, limit processed and junk food, choose healthy fats, get enough protein, take prenatal vitamins, and avoid alcohol, smoking, and drugs. By following these tips and tricks, expectant mothers can ensure a healthy and successful pregnancy. Remember to consult your healthcare provider for personalized recommendations and advice on maintaining a healthy pregnancy diet.

2. How to Exercise Safely during Pregnancy

2.1. Introduction

Pregnancy is a special time in a woman's life, and exercise can play a crucial role in maintaining a healthy pregnancy. However, exercising during pregnancy requires some caution and modification to ensure the safety 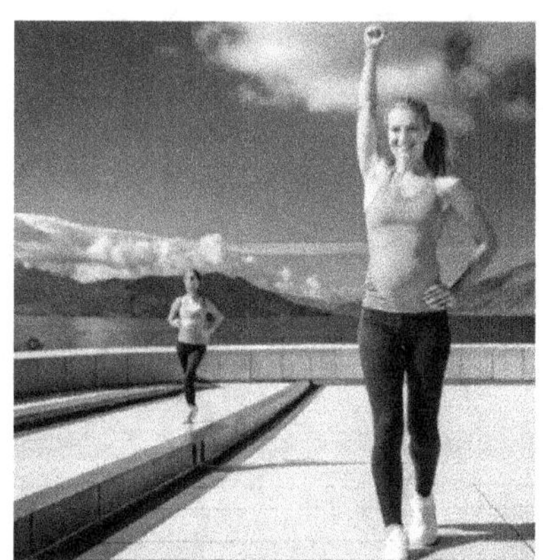 of both the mother and the developing baby. This chapter will discuss how to exercise safely during pregnancy, including real-life examples, anecdotes, helpful tips, tricks, and tools that readers can use to apply the concepts covered in the article to their own lives and situations. Before we dive into the tips for exercising safely during pregnancy, it's essential to note that every pregnancy is unique, and what works for one woman may not work for another. Therefore, it's always important to consult with your healthcare provider before starting any exercise regimen during pregnancy.

2.2. Strategies for Starting your Exercise Regimen

1. Start Slow and Gradually Increase Intensity

One of the essential tips for exercising safely during pregnancy is to start slow and gradually increase intensity. Pregnancy is not the time to push yourself to the limit or try new, intense workouts. Instead, focus on low-impact exercises, such as walking, swimming, prenatal yoga, or pilates.

Real-life example: Jane, a first-time pregnant mother, has never been into exercise before. However, she wants to start exercising to have a healthy pregnancy. Jane consulted with her healthcare provider, who recommended starting with 10 minutes of walking a day and gradually increasing to 30 minutes a day.

2. Listen to Your Body

During pregnancy, your body is going through numerous changes, and what worked for you before may not work for you now. It's essential to listen to your body and modify your exercise regimen accordingly. If something doesn't feel right, stop immediately and consult with your healthcare provider.

Real-life example: Sarah, a second-time pregnant mother, loved to run before pregnancy. However, during her second pregnancy, she noticed that running caused discomfort and pelvic pain. Sarah consulted with her healthcare provider and switched to low-impact exercises, such as swimming and prenatal yoga.

3. Stay Hydrated

Staying hydrated is crucial during pregnancy, especially when exercising. Dehydration can cause contractions, which can be dangerous for the developing baby. Make sure to drink plenty of water before, during, and after exercise.

Real-life example: Mary, a third-time pregnant mother, loved to walk outside during her pregnancy. However, she noticed that she became easily dehydrated during her walks. Mary started bringing a water bottle with her on her walks and took frequent breaks to drink water.

4. Avoid Overheating

During pregnancy, your body temperature is already elevated, and overheating can be dangerous for the developing baby. Therefore, it's important to avoid exercising in hot, humid conditions and to stay hydrated.

Real-life example: Emma, a fourth-time pregnant mother, loved to exercise outdoors during the summer months. However, she noticed that exercising outside in the heat made her feel dizzy and nauseous. Emma started exercising indoors or in the early morning or evening when the temperatures were cooler.

5. Avoid High-Risk Activities

High-risk activities, such as contact sports or activities with a high risk of falling, should be avoided during pregnancy. These activities can increase the risk of injury to both the mother and the developing baby.

Real-life example: Jenna, a fifth-time pregnant mother, loved to play soccer before pregnancy. However, she consulted with her healthcare provider and switched to low-impact exercises, such as prenatal yoga and swimming, during pregnancy.

6. Wear Proper Clothing

During pregnancy, your body is changing rapidly, and it's essential to wear comfortable, supportive clothing that allows for movement. Avoid tight-fitting clothing that restricts movement or causes discomfort.

Real-life example: Katie, a sixth-time pregnant mother, loved to exercise in her pre-pregnancy workout clothes. However, she noticed that her clothes were becoming tight and uncomfortable. Katie switched to maternity workout clothes that were designed to support her growing belly and allow for movement.

7. Modify Exercises for Your Growing Belly

As your belly grows during pregnancy, some exercises may become more difficult or uncomfortable. It's important to modify exercises to accommodate your changing body. For example, if you're doing yoga or pilates, use blocks or props to support your belly during certain poses.

Real-life example: Lisa, a seventh-time pregnant mother, loved to do yoga before pregnancy. However, as her belly grew, she found it difficult to do certain poses. Lisa consulted with her yoga instructor and modified certain poses to accommodate her growing belly.

8. Don't Overdo It

Exercise is important during pregnancy, but it's also essential to listen to your body and not overdo it. Avoid pushing yourself too hard or exercising to the point of exhaustion. Rest when needed and take breaks during exercise.

Real-life example: Rachel, an eighth-time pregnant mother, loved to walk every day during her pregnancy. However, she noticed that she was becoming easily fatigued and short of breath. Rachel started taking more breaks during her walks and resting when needed.

9. Keep Your Heart Rate in Check

During pregnancy, your heart is working harder to support the developing baby. It's important to keep your heart rate in check during exercise and not exceed a safe level. Your healthcare provider can provide guidance on what heart rate is safe for you during exercise.

Real-life example: Laura, a ninth-time pregnant mother, loved to do cardio workouts before pregnancy. However, she consulted with her healthcare provider and modified her workouts to keep her heart rate in check during pregnancy.

10.   Don't Exercise on an Empty Stomach

Exercising on an empty stomach can cause low blood sugar, which can be dangerous for both the mother and the developing baby. Eat a small snack, such as a piece of fruit or a granola bar, before exercising.

Real-life example: Megan, a tenth-time pregnant mother, loved to exercise first thing in the morning. However, she noticed that she felt lightheaded and weak during her workouts. Megan started eating a small snack before exercising to maintain her blood sugar levels.

2.3. Conclusion

Exercise is an important aspect of a healthy pregnancy, but it's crucial to exercise safely and modify your exercise regimen to accommodate your changing body. By starting slow, listening to your body, staying hydrated, avoiding overheating and high-risk activities, wearing proper clothing, modifying exercises, not overdoing it, keeping your heart rate in check, and not exercising on an empty stomach, you can exercise safely during pregnancy and have a healthy pregnancy. Remember to consult with your healthcare provider before starting any exercise regimen during pregnancy and always listen to your body.

3. How to Manage Morning Sickness during Pregnancy

3.1. Introduction

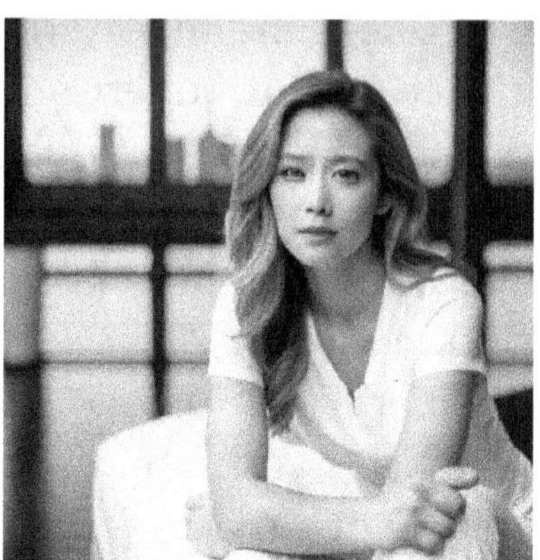

Morning sickness is a common experience during pregnancy, affecting up to 80% of expectant mothers (American College of Obstetricians and Gynecologists. (2020). Morning sickness: nausea and vomiting of pregnancy). This symptom, characterized by nausea and vomiting, can make it difficult to carry out day-to-day activities and can cause a lot of discomfort. However, with the right strategies and tools, it is possible to manage morning sickness and minimize its impact on daily life. This chapter will explore some helpful tips and tricks for managing morning sickness during pregnancy.

3.2. Strategies for Managing Morning Sickness

1. Eat Small, Frequent Meals

One of the most effective ways to manage morning sickness is to eat small, frequent meals throughout the day. Eating small amounts of food every few hours can help to keep your blood sugar levels stable and prevent nausea and vomiting. Try to choose healthy, nutrient-dense foods such as fruits, vegetables, whole grains, and lean proteins.

2. Avoid Triggers

Certain foods and smells can trigger nausea and vomiting in some women. If you notice that certain foods or smells make you feel sick, try to avoid them as much as possible. Common triggers include spicy or greasy foods, strong smells, and foods with strong flavors.

3. Stay Hydrated

Dehydration can worsen nausea and vomiting, so it is important to stay hydrated during pregnancy. Drinking water, herbal tea, and other non-caffeinated beverages can help to keep you hydrated and may also help to soothe nausea. Try sipping on fluids throughout the day instead of drinking large amounts at once.

4. Get Plenty of Rest

Fatigue can exacerbate morning sickness, so it is important to get plenty of rest during pregnancy. Aim for at least 7-8 hours of sleep per night and take naps during the day if you feel tired. If possible, try to take breaks throughout the day to rest and relax.

5. Use Aromatherapy

Aromatherapy can be a helpful tool for managing morning sickness. Scents such as peppermint, ginger, and lemon have been shown to have a calming effect and may help to soothe nausea. You can use essential oils or aromatherapy diffusers to incorporate these scents into your daily routine.

6. Try Acupressure

Acupressure is a technique that involves applying pressure to specific points on the body to alleviate symptoms. Several studies have shown that acupressure can be an effective treatment for morning sickness. You can try using acupressure bands or practicing acupressure on your own by applying pressure to the P6 point on your wrist.

7. Talk to Your Doctor

If your morning sickness is severe or is interfering with your daily life, it is important to talk to your doctor. Your doctor may be able to prescribe medications to help manage your symptoms or may recommend other treatments or lifestyle changes.

3.3. Real-Life Examples

It can be helpful to hear from other women who have experienced morning sickness and learn about the strategies that worked for them. Here are a few real-life examples:

- "I found that eating a few crackers before getting out of bed in the morning helped to settle my stomach. I kept a box of crackers on my nightstand and would eat a few as soon as I woke up."

- "I couldn't stand the smell of cooking food during my first trimester, so I made sure to eat cold foods like sandwiches and salads instead. It made a big difference in how I felt."

- "I used acupressure bands on my wrists and found that they really helped to reduce my nausea. I wore them all day, every day, and even kept a spare pair in my purse just in case."

3.4. Tricks and Tools

Here are a few additional tricks and tools that can be helpful for managing morning sickness:

- Keep a food diary to track which foods and drinks make you feel sick. This can help you to identify patterns and make adjustments to your diet.

- Use distraction techniques to take your mind off of nausea. Reading a book, listening to music, or watching a movie can all be helpful ways to distract yourself.

- Experiment with different foods and drinks to find what works best for you. Some women find that sour foods, such as lemon or lime, help to reduce nausea, while others prefer bland foods.

- Consider trying alternative therapies such as acupuncture or hypnotherapy. These techniques have been shown to be effective in managing morning sickness for some women.

- Don't be afraid to ask for help. If you are struggling with morning sickness, reach out to your partner, friends, or family members for support. They may be able to help with household tasks or offer emotional support.

3.5. Conclusion

Morning sickness can be a challenging symptom to manage during pregnancy, but with the right strategies and tools, it is possible to minimize its impact on daily life. Eating small, frequent meals, avoiding triggers, staying hydrated, getting plenty of rest, using aromatherapy and acupressure, and talking to your doctor are all helpful ways to manage morning sickness. Real-life examples and additional tricks and tools can also be useful for finding what works best for you. Remember to be patient with yourself and to reach out for help when needed. With the right support, you can manage morning sickness and enjoy a healthy pregnancy.

4. How to Deal with Pregnancy-related Back Pain

4.1. Introduction

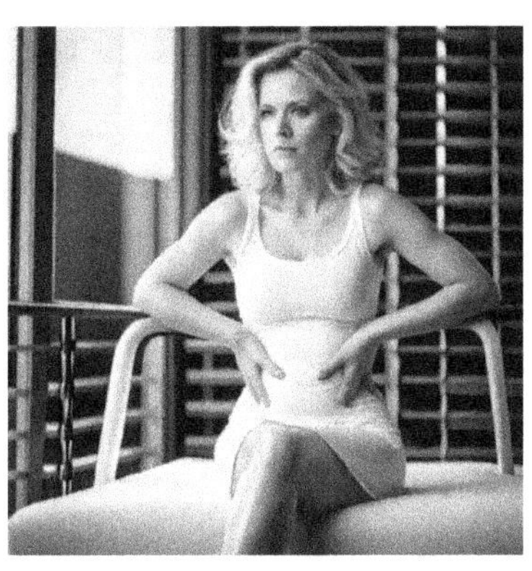

Pregnancy is an exciting and beautiful time in a woman's life, but it can also be quite challenging. One of the most common challenges faced by pregnant women is pregnancy-related back pain. As the baby grows, the mother's center of gravity shifts, causing the muscles and ligaments in the back to stretch and strain. This can result in a variety of uncomfortable symptoms, such as stiffness, soreness, and even sharp pains. This chapter will explore some of the best ways to deal with pregnancy-related back pain and make this special time as comfortable as possible.

4.2. Best Ways for Dealing with Pregnancy-Related Back Pain

1. Practice Good Posture

One of the simplest but most effective ways to reduce pregnancy-related back pain is to practice good posture. When standing, make sure your shoulders are relaxed, your chest is lifted, and your weight is evenly distributed on both feet. Avoid locking your knees and tucking your tailbone under, as this can strain the lower back. When sitting, choose a chair with good back support and use a small pillow or rolled-up towel to support the curve of your lower back.

2. Exercise Regularly

Regular exercise during pregnancy can help alleviate back pain and other discomforts. Low-impact exercises such as walking, swimming, and yoga are excellent choices for pregnant women. These activities help improve flexibility, strengthen muscles, and improve circulation, which can all help reduce back pain. Be sure to consult with your healthcare provider before starting any exercise program during pregnancy.

3. Use Heat or Cold Therapy

Heat or cold therapy can be a helpful tool for reducing pregnancy-related back pain. Applying a heating pad or warm towel to the affected area can help relax muscles and increase circulation, while a cold pack can reduce inflammation and numb pain. Try alternating between hot and cold therapy to find what works best for you.

4. Get a Massage

A prenatal massage from a licensed massage therapist can be a wonderful way to relieve back pain and promote relaxation. A skilled therapist will know how to work with the unique needs of pregnant women and can use techniques such as gentle stretching and pressure point massage to alleviate tension and soreness in the back.

5. Wear Supportive Shoes

Wearing supportive shoes can make a big difference in reducing pregnancy-related back pain. Look for shoes with good arch support, a cushioned sole, and a low heel. Avoid high heels, as they can strain the lower back and alter your posture.

6. Practice Relaxation Techniques

Stress and tension can exacerbate back pain during pregnancy, so practicing relaxation techniques such as deep breathing, meditation, or visualization can be very helpful. Try to find a quiet and peaceful space where you can sit or lie down comfortably, close your eyes, and focus on your breath or a calming mental image.

7. Use a Support Belt

A support belt can provide extra support to the lower back and relieve pressure on the pelvis. These belts are designed to be worn low on the hips and can be adjusted to provide the right amount of support. They can be especially helpful in the later stages of pregnancy when the baby's weight is putting more strain on the back and pelvis.

8. Try Acupuncture

Acupuncture is an ancient Chinese healing practice that involves inserting thin needles into specific points on the body. It is believed to stimulate the body's natural healing processes and can be an effective way to relieve back pain during pregnancy. Be sure to find a licensed and experienced acupuncturist who is trained to work with pregnant women.

9. Use a Pregnancy Pillow

A pregnancy pillow is a specially designed pillow that can help support the body during sleep. It can help alleviate back pain by providing support to the hips, back, and belly, which can help take pressure off the spine. There are many different types of pregnancy pillows available, so be sure to choose one that fits your needs and sleeping preferences.

10.   Consult with a Healthcare Provider

If you are experiencing persistent or severe back pain during pregnancy, it is important to consult with your healthcare provider. They can help diagnose the underlying cause of the pain and recommend appropriate treatments or therapies. In some cases, more serious conditions such as sciatica or herniated discs may be causing the pain, and medical intervention may be necessary.

4.3. Real-life Examples

Many women experience pregnancy-related back pain, and it can be a challenging symptom to manage. However, with the right strategies and tools, it is possible to reduce discomfort and enjoy a more comfortable pregnancy.

One expectant mother, Jane, found that regular exercise and yoga helped alleviate her back pain during pregnancy. She joined a prenatal yoga class and found that the gentle stretching and relaxation techniques helped reduce tension and soreness in her back.

Another mother, Sarah, found that using a pregnancy pillow made a big difference in her comfort level during sleep. She chose a U-shaped pillow that provided support to her hips, back, and belly, and she found that it helped reduce pressure on her spine and reduce back pain.

4.4. Tricks and Tools

In addition to the strategies listed above, there are a few other tricks and tools that can be helpful for managing pregnancy-related back pain. These include:

- Using a foam roller to massage sore muscles

- Taking warm baths or showers to relax the body

- Practicing pelvic tilts to strengthen the muscles in the lower back and abdomen

- Avoiding standing or sitting for long periods of time without taking breaks to move around and stretch

4.5. Conclusion

Pregnancy-related back pain is a common and often uncomfortable symptom of pregnancy. However, there are many strategies and tools that can help reduce discomfort and promote relaxation during this special time. By practicing good posture, exercising regularly, using heat or cold therapy, getting a massage, wearing supportive shoes, practicing relaxation techniques, using a support belt, trying acupuncture, using a pregnancy pillow, and consulting with a healthcare provider, women can manage pregnancy-related back pain and enjoy a more comfortable pregnancy.

5. How to Cope With Pregnancy-Related Anxiety

5.1. Introduction

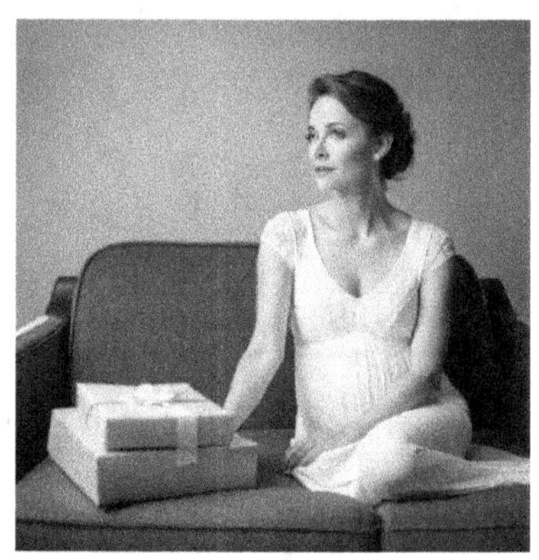

Pregnancy is an exciting time for many women, but it can also be a time of great anxiety. With so many physical and emotional changes happening in the body, it's normal to feel anxious and overwhelmed. However, pregnancy-related anxiety can be managed with the right tools and support. This chapter will explore some helpful tips and tricks for coping with pregnancy-related anxiety.

5.2. Strategies for Coping with Pregnancy-Related Anxiety

1. Educate Yourself

One of the best ways to cope with pregnancy-related anxiety is to educate yourself about what to expect during pregnancy. Learn about the physical and emotional changes that occur during each trimester. Understanding the changes happening in your body and how they affect you can help alleviate anxiety. It is also helpful to learn about the signs and symptoms of pregnancy-related complications, such as pre-eclampsia, gestational diabetes, or placenta previa. Knowing what to look for and when to seek medical attention can help alleviate anxiety.

2. Communicate with Your Healthcare Provider

Communication with your healthcare provider is essential during pregnancy. Don't be afraid to ask questions and express your concerns. Your healthcare provider can provide reassurance, guidance, and support. They can also refer you to mental health professionals or support groups if necessary.

3. Connect with Other Pregnant Women

Connecting with other pregnant women can provide a sense of community and support. You can join pregnancy support groups or attend prenatal classes. Sharing experiences and feelings with other women who are going through the same thing can be reassuring.

4. Practice Relaxation Techniques

Practicing relaxation techniques can help alleviate anxiety. Techniques such as deep breathing, meditation, and yoga can help calm the mind and body. These techniques can also improve sleep, reduce stress, and promote overall wellbeing.

5. Exercise Regularly

Exercise during pregnancy is safe and beneficial for both you and your baby. Exercise can improve mood, reduce stress, and increase energy levels. It can also help alleviate anxiety by releasing endorphins, which are natural mood boosters.

6. Maintain a Healthy Diet

A healthy diet is important during pregnancy. Eating a variety of fruits, vegetables, whole grains, and lean protein can provide the necessary nutrients for a healthy pregnancy. Avoiding caffeine, alcohol, and processed foods can also improve overall health and wellbeing.

7. Get Enough Sleep

Getting enough sleep is crucial during pregnancy. Sleep deprivation can exacerbate anxiety symptoms. Aim for 7-9 hours of sleep per night. If you're having trouble sleeping, try relaxation techniques or talk to your healthcare provider about sleep aids.

8. Plan Ahead

Planning ahead can help alleviate anxiety. Create a birth plan, prepare the baby's nursery, and plan for maternity leave. Having a plan in place can provide a sense of control and reduce anxiety.

9. Talk to Your Partner

Talking to your partner about your feelings can provide emotional support. Your partner can offer reassurance, comfort, and help alleviate anxiety. Don't be afraid to ask for help or support when you need it.

10. Seek Professional Help

If pregnancy-related anxiety becomes overwhelming, seeking professional help is essential. Mental health professionals can provide therapy and medication if necessary. Talk to your healthcare provider about mental health resources in your area.

5.3. Real-Life Examples

Pregnancy-related anxiety is a common experience for many women. Here are some real-life examples and anecdotes from women who have experienced pregnancy-related anxiety.

- ✓ "I was worried about everything during my pregnancy. I worried about the health of my baby, the delivery, and being a good mother. Talking to my healthcare provider and joining a support group helped alleviate my anxiety. I also practiced relaxation techniques and exercised regularly, which helped improve my mood."

- ✓ "I had a high-risk pregnancy, and I was anxious about complications. My healthcare provider referred me to a mental health professional, who provided therapy and medication. Talking to someone who understood my fears and concerns was incredibly helpful. It also gave me tools to manage my anxiety, which helped me enjoy my pregnancy more."

- ✓ "I struggled with insomnia during my pregnancy, which made my anxiety worse. My healthcare provider recommended sleep aids, but I was hesitant to take medication. Instead, I tried relaxation techniques, such as deep breathing and meditation, and they worked wonders. I was able to get better sleep and reduce my anxiety without medication."

5.4. Tricks and Tools

Here are some additional tricks and tools for coping with pregnancy-related anxiety:

1. Write in a Journal

Writing in a journal can be a helpful tool for managing anxiety. Write down your thoughts and feelings, and try to identify any patterns or triggers. This can help you understand your anxiety and develop coping strategies.

2. Create a Gratitude List

Creating a gratitude list can help shift your focus from anxiety to gratitude. Write down three things you're grateful for each day. This can help cultivate a more positive mindset and reduce anxiety.

3. Practice Mindfulness

Mindfulness involves being present in the moment and accepting your thoughts and feelings without judgment. Mindfulness can be practiced through meditation, yoga, or simply taking a few deep breaths. Practicing mindfulness can help reduce anxiety and improve overall wellbeing.

4. Use Positive Affirmations

Positive affirmations are statements that promote positive self-talk. Repeat positive affirmations to yourself throughout the day, such as "I am capable of handling whatever comes my way" or "My body is strong and capable of giving birth." Positive affirmations can help promote self-confidence and reduce anxiety.

5. Take Breaks

Taking breaks throughout the day can help reduce stress and anxiety. Take a walk, read a book, or listen to music. Giving yourself permission to take breaks can help alleviate anxiety and improve productivity.

5.5. Conclusion

Pregnancy-related anxiety is a common experience, but it can be managed with the right tools and support. Educate yourself about pregnancy, communicate with your healthcare provider, connect with other pregnant women, practice relaxation techniques, exercise regularly, maintain a healthy diet, get enough sleep, plan ahead, talk to your partner, and seek professional help if necessary. Remember, pregnancy is a time of great change and transformation, and it is okay to feel anxious. With the right tools and support, you can cope with pregnancy-related anxiety and enjoy this special time in your life.

6. How to Avoid and Manage Gestational Diabetes

6.1. Introduction

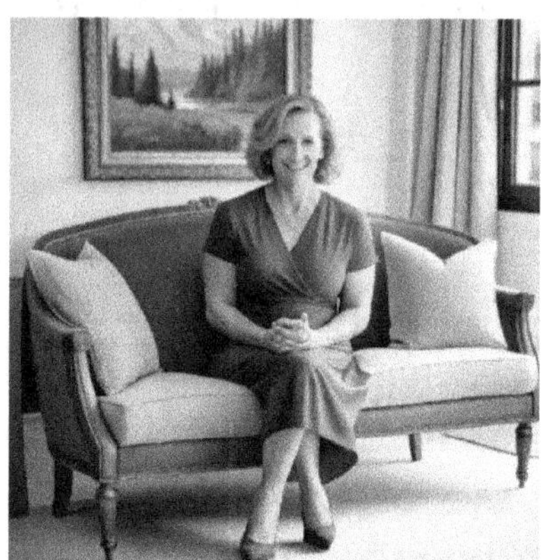

Gestational diabetes is a type of diabetes that develops during pregnancy. It is a condition that affects many women during pregnancy and can cause serious health problems for both mother and baby. The good news is that there are ways to avoid and manage gestational diabetes, and with some careful planning and lifestyle changes, you can reduce your risk and keep yourself and your baby healthy.

6.2. What is gestational diabetes?

Gestational diabetes is a type of diabetes that develops during pregnancy. It occurs when the body is unable to produce enough insulin to regulate the sugar levels in the blood. The condition is more common in women who are overweight or have a family history of diabetes. It can also be caused by a lack of exercise or poor diet.

6.3. Symptoms of gestational diabetes

The symptoms of gestational diabetes can be similar to those of other types of diabetes. They can include:

- Feeling thirsty

- Needing to urinate more often

- Feeling tired or weak

- Blurred vision

- Feeling dizzy or light-headed

However, many women with gestational diabetes do not experience any symptoms, which is why it is important to be screened for the condition during pregnancy.

6.4. How to avoid gestational diabetes

The best way to avoid gestational diabetes is to maintain a healthy weight and lifestyle before and during pregnancy. Here are some tips to help you reduce your risk:

1. Eat a healthy diet

Eating a healthy and balanced diet is important for both you and your baby. Try to include plenty of fruits, vegetables, whole grains, lean proteins, and healthy fats in your diet. Avoid processed foods and sugary drinks, as these can increase your risk of developing gestational diabetes.

2. Exercise regularly

Regular exercise can help you maintain a healthy weight and reduce your risk of developing gestational diabetes. Try to aim for at least 30 minutes of moderate exercise, such as walking or swimming, most days of the week. Always check with your doctor before starting a new exercise program.

3. Manage stress

Stress can affect your blood sugar levels, so it is important to manage it as much as possible. Try to practice relaxation techniques such as deep breathing or yoga, and find ways to reduce stress in your daily life.

4. Get screened

All pregnant women should be screened for gestational diabetes between 24 and 28 weeks of pregnancy. If you are at higher risk, your doctor may recommend earlier screening.

6.5. How to manage gestational diabetes

If you are diagnosed with gestational diabetes, there are several things you can do to manage the condition and keep yourself and your baby healthy. Here are some tips:

1. Follow a healthy diet

Following a healthy diet is crucial for managing gestational diabetes. Your doctor or a registered dietitian can help you create a meal plan that is tailored to your needs. This may involve limiting your intake of carbohydrates and sugars, and focusing on lean proteins, fruits, vegetables, and whole grains.

2. Exercise regularly

Regular exercise can help you control your blood sugar levels and manage gestational diabetes. Aim for at least 30 minutes of moderate exercise, such as walking or swimming, most days of the week. Always check with your doctor before starting a new exercise program.

3. Monitor your blood sugar levels

You will need to monitor your blood sugar levels regularly during pregnancy. Your doctor will show you how to use a glucose meter to check your levels at home. Keeping a record of your blood sugar levels can help you and your doctor adjust your treatment plan as needed.

4. Take medication if needed

In some cases, medication may be needed to control gestational diabetes. Your doctor may prescribe insulin or other medications to help manage your blood sugar levels. It is important to follow your doctor's instructions and take your medication as prescribed.

5. Attend regular check-ups

Attending regular check-ups is an important part of managing gestational diabetes. Your healthcare team will monitor your blood sugar levels, check the growth and development of your baby, and make any necessary adjustments to your treatment plan. During your check-ups, your healthcare team may also perform additional tests to monitor your condition, such as a fetal ultrasound to check your baby's growth or a non-stress test to monitor your baby's heart rate. It is important to attend all scheduled check-ups and follow any recommendations or instructions from your healthcare team. If you have any questions or concerns, don't hesitate to ask your doctor or diabetes educator for advice. They are there to support you throughout your pregnancy and ensure the best possible outcome for you and your baby. In addition to the above tips, there are some other things you can do to manage gestational diabetes and keep yourself and your baby healthy:

1. Stay hydrated

Drinking plenty of water can help regulate your blood sugar levels and prevent dehydration. Aim for at least 8-10 glasses of water per day.

2. Get enough sleep

Getting enough sleep is important for overall health and can help regulate blood sugar levels. Aim for 7-8 hours of sleep per night, and try to establish a regular sleep routine.

3. Manage stress

Stress can affect blood sugar levels, so it is important to find ways to manage stress during pregnancy. This may include practicing relaxation techniques such as deep breathing or yoga, or finding ways to reduce stress in your daily life.

4. Stay in touch with your healthcare team

Your healthcare team will be monitoring your progress and helping you manage your gestational diabetes. It is important to attend all scheduled check-ups and follow their recommendations for managing your condition.

6.6. Real-life examples

Managing gestational diabetes can be challenging, but with the right support and resources, it is possible to keep yourself and your baby healthy. Here are some real-life examples of women who successfully managed their gestational diabetes:

- Sarah was diagnosed with gestational diabetes during her second trimester. She worked with a registered dietitian to create a meal plan that was tailored to her needs and monitored her blood sugar levels regularly. With these lifestyle changes and medication, she was able to keep her blood sugar levels in check and deliver a healthy baby.

- Maria had a family history of diabetes and was at higher risk of developing gestational diabetes. She focused on maintaining a healthy weight and eating a balanced diet before and during pregnancy. She also stayed active by walking and practicing yoga. She was screened for gestational diabetes at 24 weeks and was relieved to find out she did not have the condition.

6.7. Tools and resources

There are many tools and resources available to help you manage gestational diabetes. Here are some examples:

- **Glucose meter:** A glucose meter is a small device that allows you to check your blood sugar levels at home. Your doctor or diabetes educator can show you how to use it.

- **Meal planning tools:** There are many meal planning tools and apps available that can help you create a healthy and balanced meal plan. Some examples include MyFitnessPal and SparkPeople.

- **Support groups:** Joining a support group for women with gestational diabetes can provide you with valuable support and resources. You can ask your healthcare team for recommendations or search online for groups in your area.

6.8. Conclusion

Gestational diabetes is a common condition that affects many women during pregnancy. While it can be challenging to manage, there are many things you can do to reduce your risk and keep yourself and your baby healthy. By following a healthy diet, staying active, monitoring your blood sugar levels, and getting support from your healthcare team, you can successfully manage gestational diabetes and have a healthy pregnancy. Remember to stay in touch with your healthcare team and follow their recommendations for managing your condition.

7. How to Manage Fatigue during Pregnancy

7.1. Introduction

Pregnancy is an exciting time, but it can also be a tiring one. As your body goes through significant changes, fatigue can become a common symptom. Managing fatigue during pregnancy can be challenging, but with the right 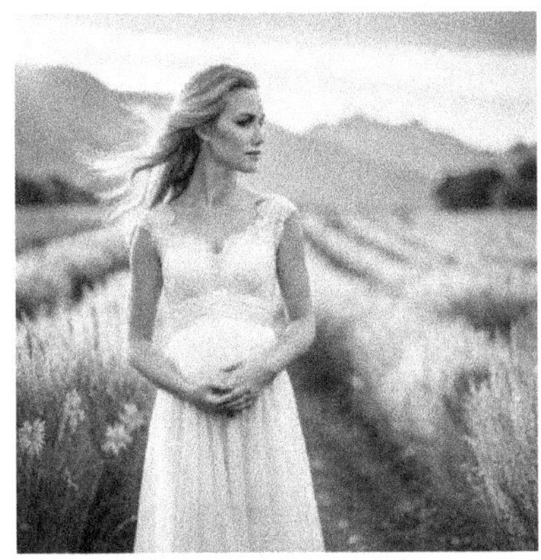 strategies, you can ensure you stay healthy, energetic, and productive throughout this beautiful journey. This chapter will discuss helpful tips, tricks, and tools to manage fatigue during pregnancy. Let's dive in!

7.2. Strategies for Managing Fatigue during Pregnancy

1. Get Enough Rest

Rest is essential during pregnancy, and getting enough sleep is crucial for combating fatigue. Try to get at least eight hours of sleep per night, and if possible, take a nap during the day. Listen to your body and allow yourself to rest when you feel tired.

2. Stay Active

Although it may be tempting to rest all day, exercise can help reduce fatigue during pregnancy. Low-impact activities such as walking, yoga, and swimming can boost energy levels and help you sleep better at night. Be sure to consult your healthcare provider before starting any new exercise regimen.

3. Stay Hydrated

Staying hydrated is vital during pregnancy as dehydration can cause fatigue. Drink plenty of water throughout the day, and avoid caffeinated or sugary beverages as they can dehydrate you.

4. Eat a Healthy Diet

Eating a healthy, balanced diet can help keep your energy levels up. Choose nutrient-dense foods such as fruits, vegetables, lean proteins, and whole grains. Avoid processed foods, sugary snacks, and drinks as they can cause energy crashes.

5. Take Breaks

Pregnancy can be exhausting, and taking breaks throughout the day can help manage fatigue. Take short breaks during work or household tasks, and allow yourself to rest whenever you need it.

6. Ask for Help

Don't be afraid to ask for help from friends, family, or your partner. They can help with household tasks or childcare, giving you time to rest and recharge.

7. Prioritize Self-Care

Taking care of yourself is essential during pregnancy, and self-care practices can help combat fatigue. Try activities such as meditation, yoga, or a warm bath to help you relax and recharge.

8. Manage Stress

Stress can cause fatigue during pregnancy, so it's essential to manage it effectively. Try relaxation techniques such as deep breathing or mindfulness meditation to reduce stress levels.

7.3. Real-life examples, Anecdotes, and Tools

Real-life examples

"I was exhausted during my first trimester and found it challenging to manage fatigue. I started taking short naps during the day and reduced my work hours to manage my energy levels. I also started eating a healthier diet, and that made a big difference in my energy levels."

Anecdotes

"My wife experienced severe fatigue during her third trimester, and it was challenging for her to manage it. We started taking walks together every day, and that helped boost her energy levels. We also made sure she got enough rest and took breaks throughout the day."

Tools

1. A pregnancy journal can help you track your energy levels, sleep patterns, and exercise routines. This can help you identify patterns and make adjustments to manage fatigue effectively.

2. A pregnancy pillow can help you get comfortable during sleep and reduce discomfort, allowing you to get better quality sleep.

3. A fitness tracker can help you track your exercise routine and monitor your progress. This can motivate you to stay active and help you manage fatigue effectively.

4. A mindfulness app can help you manage stress levels and promote relaxation. Apps such as Headspace and Calm offer guided meditations and breathing exercises designed to help you manage stress.

5. A meal planner can help you plan healthy, balanced meals and ensure you're getting the nutrients you need to manage fatigue. Apps such as Mealime and Meal Planner Pro offer customizable meal plans and grocery lists to make meal planning easy.

7.4. Conclusion

Managing fatigue during pregnancy can be challenging, but with the right strategies, it is possible to combat this common symptom effectively. It's essential to prioritize rest, exercise, hydration, and a healthy diet, as well as taking breaks, asking for help, and prioritizing self-care.

Remember to listen to your body and give yourself permission to rest when you need it. Don't be afraid to ask for help, and consider using tools such as pregnancy journals, pregnancy pillows, fitness trackers, mindfulness apps, and meal planners to help you manage fatigue effectively.

It's important to note that fatigue can be a sign of underlying health issues, so if your fatigue is severe, persistent, or accompanied by other symptoms, be sure to speak with your healthcare provider. They can help identify any underlying health issues and provide appropriate treatment. Overall, managing fatigue during pregnancy requires a combination of lifestyle changes, self-care practices, and the use of helpful tools and resources. With the right strategies, you can stay healthy, energetic, and productive throughout your pregnancy, ensuring you and your baby have a happy and healthy journey.

8.   How to Deal with Pregnancy-related Insomnia

8.1. Introduction

Pregnancy is an exciting and transformative time, but it can also come with a host of physical and emotional challenges, including insomnia. Up to 78% of women report trouble sleeping during pregnancy, especially in the third 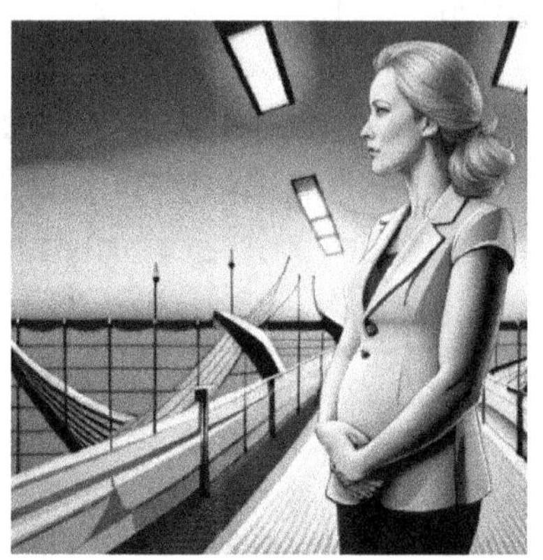 trimester (Sleep Medicine Reviews in 2018). The good news is that there are plenty of strategies you can use to manage pregnancy-related insomnia and get the rest you need.

8.2. What causes pregnancy-related insomnia?

There are a few reasons why pregnant women may experience insomnia. Firstly, hormonal changes can impact sleep patterns, especially in the first and third trimesters. Secondly, physical discomfort, such as back pain, heartburn, and frequent urination, can make it difficult to get comfortable enough to fall asleep and stay asleep. Finally, anxiety and stress related to pregnancy and impending motherhood can also keep you up at night.

8.3. Tips for managing pregnancy-related insomnia

1. Establish a bedtime routine

Creating a consistent bedtime routine can help signal to your body that it's time to wind down and prepare for sleep. Your routine can include activities such as taking a warm bath, reading a book, or doing some gentle stretches or relaxation exercises. Whatever you choose, make sure it's relaxing and enjoyable for you.

2. Make your bedroom a sleep-friendly environment

Your bedroom should be a sanctuary for sleep, free from distractions and stimuli that could interfere with your rest. Consider investing in blackout curtains, a white noise machine, or comfortable bedding to create a calm and peaceful environment. Keeping your bedroom cool and well-ventilated can also help promote sleep.

3. Practice good sleep hygiene

Good sleep hygiene habits can help regulate your sleep-wake cycle and promote better sleep quality. These habits include going to bed and waking up at the same time each day, avoiding napping during the day, limiting caffeine and alcohol intake, and avoiding screen time for at least an hour before bed.

4. Manage physical discomfort

If physical discomfort is keeping you awake, there are a few things you can do to manage it. Experiment with different sleeping positions, such as sleeping on your side with a pillow between your legs or using a pregnancy pillow to support your belly and back. You can also try using a heating pad or taking a warm bath before bed to ease muscle tension.

5. Address anxiety and stress

If anxiety or stress related to pregnancy or impending motherhood is interfering with your sleep, it's important to address it. Consider talking to a therapist or counselor who can help you develop coping strategies and provide emotional support. You can also try relaxation techniques such as deep breathing, meditation, or visualization to calm your mind and body.

6. Stay active

Staying active during pregnancy can help regulate your sleep-wake cycle and promote better sleep quality. However, it's important to avoid strenuous exercise close to bedtime, as this can actually make it harder to fall asleep. Instead, aim to exercise earlier in the day and incorporate gentle activities such as prenatal yoga or walking into your routine.

7. Try natural remedies

There are several natural remedies that may help promote relaxation and sleep, such as chamomile tea, lavender essential oil, and valerian root. However, it's important to talk to your healthcare provider before using any herbal supplements or remedies during pregnancy, as some may not be safe for you or your baby.

8.4. Real-life examples

Jenna, a first-time mother, struggled with pregnancy-related insomnia throughout her entire pregnancy. She tried several strategies, including establishing a consistent bedtime routine, creating a sleep-friendly environment, and managing physical discomfort. However, she found that her anxiety about becoming a mother continued to keep her up at night. Eventually, she decided to seek the help of a therapist who specialized in perinatal mental health. Through therapy, she was able to develop coping strategies and address her anxieties, which allowed her to finally get the rest she needed.

Another mother, Rachel, found that incorporating gentle exercise into her routine, such as walking and prenatal yoga, helped her manage pregnancy-related insomnia. She also used a pregnancy pillow to support her belly and back while sleeping, which helped alleviate physical discomfort.

8.5. Tricks and tools

In addition to the tips mentioned above, there are a few tricks and tools that can help you manage pregnancy-related insomnia. Here are some ideas to consider:

1. **Use a white noise machine or app:** White noise can help drown out distracting sounds and promote relaxation. Consider using a white noise machine or

app to create a calming background noise in your bedroom.

2. **Invest in comfortable bedding:** Comfortable bedding can make a big difference in your sleep quality. Consider investing in a supportive mattress, soft sheets, and a cozy blanket to help you get comfortable and stay asleep.

3. **Keep a journal:** If anxiety or stress is keeping you up at night, consider keeping a journal to express your thoughts and feelings. Writing down your worries can help you process them and release some of the tension and stress you may be carrying.

4. **Try progressive muscle relaxation:** Progressive muscle relaxation is a relaxation technique that involves tensing and releasing each muscle group in your body. This can help release muscle tension and promote relaxation throughout your body.

5. **Consider a pregnancy sleep program:** There are several pregnancy sleep programs available online that provide guidance and support for managing pregnancy-related insomnia. These programs may include personalized sleep plans, coaching, and educational resources to help you get the rest you need.

8.6. Conclusion

Pregnancy-related insomnia is a common and challenging issue for many expectant mothers. However, there are plenty of strategies you can use to manage your sleep and get the rest you need. By establishing a consistent bedtime routine, creating a sleep-friendly environment, managing physical discomfort, addressing anxiety and stress, staying active, and trying natural remedies, you can improve your sleep quality and feel more rested and rejuvenated throughout your pregnancy. If you continue to struggle with insomnia despite trying these strategies, don't hesitate to talk to your healthcare provider, who can provide additional support and resources to help you sleep better.

9.1. Introduction

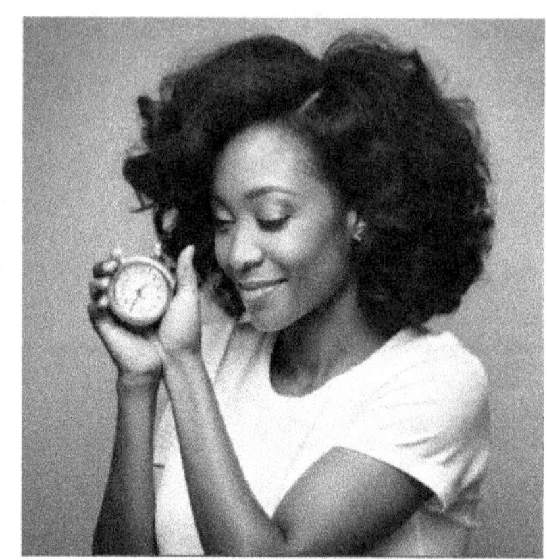

High blood pressure, also known as hypertension, is a common condition that affects many people worldwide. However, when it occurs during pregnancy, it can be particularly concerning. High blood pressure during pregnancy can lead to serious complications for both the mother and the baby. Therefore, it is essential to recognize and manage high blood pressure during pregnancy promptly. This chapter will discuss how to recognize and manage high blood pressure during pregnancy, including helpful tips, real-life examples, anecdotes, tricks, and tools that readers can use to apply the concepts covered in the article to their own lives and situations.

9.2. What is high blood pressure during pregnancy?

High blood pressure during pregnancy is defined as a systolic blood pressure (the top number) of 140 mm Hg or higher and/or a diastolic blood pressure (the bottom number) of 90 mm Hg or higher (National Heart, Lung, and Blood Institute. (2021). High blood pressure in pregnancy). High blood pressure can occur at any time during pregnancy, but it is most common after 20 weeks of gestation. High blood pressure during pregnancy can lead to serious complications, including preeclampsia, a potentially life-threatening condition that affects both the mother and the baby.

9.3. How to recognize high blood pressure during pregnancy?

Recognizing high blood pressure during pregnancy is essential to ensure timely management and prevent complications. Some common signs and symptoms of high blood pressure during pregnancy include:

a) Severe headaches
b) Blurred vision
c) Swelling in the face, hands, and feet
d) Rapid weight gain
e) Shortness of breath
f) Nausea or vomiting
g) Decreased urine output
h) Upper abdominal pain

If you experience any of these symptoms, it is crucial to contact your healthcare provider immediately.

9.4. How to manage high blood pressure during pregnancy?

Managing high blood pressure during pregnancy is essential to prevent complications and ensure the health of both the mother and the baby. Here are some tips for managing high blood pressure during pregnancy:

1. **Regular prenatal care:** Regular prenatal care is essential to monitor your blood pressure and detect

any changes or abnormalities. Your healthcare provider may recommend more frequent visits and testing to monitor your blood pressure and other vital signs.

2. **Medications:** Your healthcare provider may prescribe medication to manage your blood pressure if it is consistently high. It is essential to follow your healthcare provider's instructions regarding medication dosage and timing.

3. **Lifestyle changes:** Lifestyle changes can help manage high blood pressure during pregnancy. Some of these changes include:

   a. Eating a healthy diet rich in fruits, vegetables, and whole grains.

   b. Reducing salt intake.

   c. Staying physically active with low-impact exercises, such as walking or swimming.

   d. Managing stress through relaxation techniques, such as meditation or yoga.

   e. Avoiding smoking and alcohol consumption.

4. **Bed rest:** In some cases, your healthcare provider may recommend bed rest to manage high blood pressure during pregnancy. Bed rest can help reduce stress on your body and lower your blood pressure.

5. **Delivery:** In severe cases of high blood pressure or preeclampsia, your healthcare provider may

recommend delivery to prevent complications. Delivery may occur earlier than expected, but your healthcare provider will carefully monitor the baby's development and make recommendations based on the baby's health.

9.5. Real-life examples

Managing high blood pressure during pregnancy can be challenging, but it is possible with the right strategies and support. Here are some real-life examples and anecdotes that illustrate the importance of recognizing and managing high blood pressure during pregnancy:

1. **Sarah's story:** Sarah was 34 weeks pregnant when she started experiencing severe headaches and blurred vision. She visited her healthcare provider, who diagnosed her with preeclampsia. Sarah's healthcare provider recommended immediate hospitalization and delivery to prevent complications. Sarah gave birth to a healthy baby girl, who required a short stay in the neonatal intensive care unit for monitoring. Sarah's healthcare team closely monitored her blood pressure and other vital signs and provided appropriate medication and care to manage her condition. With regular follow-up care, Sarah and her baby both recovered well.

2. **Maria's story:** Maria was diagnosed with high blood pressure during her first trimester of pregnancy. She followed her healthcare provider's recommendations for lifestyle changes, including eating a healthy diet and staying physically active. Despite her best efforts,

Maria's blood pressure remained high, and her healthcare provider prescribed medication to manage her condition. Maria took her medication as directed and attended all her prenatal appointments for monitoring. She delivered a healthy baby boy at 39 weeks without any complications.

9.6. Helpful Tools and Tricks

Managing high blood pressure during pregnancy can be challenging, but there are some helpful tools and tricks that can make it easier. Here are some examples:

1. **Blood pressure monitor:** A blood pressure monitor can help you monitor your blood pressure at home between prenatal appointments. Your healthcare provider can recommend a suitable monitor and teach you how to use it correctly.

2. **Mobile apps:** There are several mobile apps available that can help you track your blood pressure, diet, and exercise routine. These apps can help you stay motivated and on track with your goals.

3. **Support groups:** Joining a support group for women with high blood pressure during pregnancy can provide you with valuable information and emotional support. You can share your experiences and learn from other women who have gone through similar experiences.

9.7. Conclusion

Recognizing and managing high blood pressure during pregnancy is essential to ensure the health of both the mother and the baby. Regular prenatal care, medication, lifestyle changes, bed rest, and delivery may be necessary to manage high blood pressure during pregnancy. Real-life examples and anecdotes demonstrate the importance of timely and appropriate care. Finally, using helpful tools and tricks can make managing high blood pressure during pregnancy more manageable. Remember, if you experience any symptoms of high blood pressure during pregnancy, contact your healthcare provider immediately.

10. How to Maintain a Healthy Weight during Pregnancy

10.1.   Introduction

Pregnancy is a time of great excitement and anticipation for most women. However, it can also be a time of confusion and anxiety when it comes to weight gain. While it is important to gain weight during pregnancy, excessive weight gain can lead 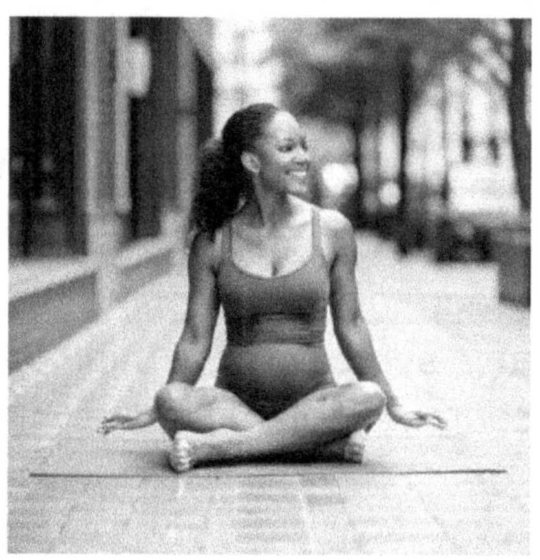 to health problems for both the mother and the baby. This chapter will discuss how to maintain a healthy weight during pregnancy by offering helpful tips, real-life examples, anecdotes, tricks, and tools that readers can use to apply the concepts covered in the article to their own lives and situations.

10.2.   Tip #1: Eat a Balanced Diet

Eating a balanced diet during pregnancy is essential for maintaining a healthy weight. A balanced diet includes a variety of fruits, vegetables, whole grains, lean protein, and healthy fats. These foods provide essential nutrients for both the mother and the baby. Additionally, eating a balanced diet can help to prevent excessive weight gain. It is important to avoid processed foods, sugary drinks, and high-fat foods during pregnancy. These foods are high in calories and can lead to weight gain.

Real-life Example: Emily is a pregnant woman who is committed to eating a balanced diet. She starts her day with a bowl of oatmeal topped with fresh berries and almond butter. For lunch, she enjoys a salad with mixed greens, grilled chicken, and a variety of vegetables. For dinner, she makes roasted salmon with quinoa and roasted vegetables. She snacks on fresh fruit, Greek yogurt, and nuts throughout the day.

Trick: Keep healthy snacks on hand. It is important to have healthy snacks on hand during pregnancy. This can help to prevent overeating and keep cravings in check. Some healthy snack options include fresh fruit, raw vegetables with hummus, Greek yogurt, and nuts.

10.3.   Tip #2: Exercise Regularly

Exercise is an important part of maintaining a healthy weight during pregnancy. Regular exercise can help to prevent excessive weight gain and improve overall health. Additionally, exercise can help to reduce the risk of gestational diabetes and other pregnancy-related complications. It is important to consult with a healthcare provider before starting an exercise routine during pregnancy.

Real-life Example: Sarah is a pregnant woman who enjoys exercising regularly. She goes for a 30-minute walk every day and attends prenatal yoga classes twice a week. She also incorporates strength training exercises into her routine to help maintain muscle tone and prevent muscle loss.

Trick: Find an exercise buddy. Having an exercise buddy can be a great way to stay motivated during pregnancy. It is important to find someone who is also committed to maintaining a healthy weight during pregnancy.

10.4. Tip #3: Monitor Weight Gain

Monitoring weight gain during pregnancy is essential for maintaining a healthy weight. While weight gain is a normal part of pregnancy, excessive weight gain can lead to health problems. It is important to discuss weight gain with a healthcare provider and monitor weight regularly.

Real-life Example: Lisa is a pregnant woman who is monitoring her weight gain carefully. She weighs herself once a week and keeps a record of her weight gain. She discusses her weight gain with her healthcare provider at each prenatal appointment.

Trick: Use a food journal. Keeping a food journal can be a great way to monitor food intake and prevent overeating. It is important to write down everything that is eaten, including portion sizes.

10.5. Tip #4: Drink Plenty of Water

Drinking plenty of water during pregnancy is essential for maintaining a healthy weight. Water helps to flush out toxins and prevent dehydration. Additionally, drinking water can help to reduce cravings for sugary drinks and other unhealthy beverages.

Real-life Example: Maria is a pregnant woman who drinks plenty of water throughout the day. She carries a reusable water bottle with her at all times and sets reminders to drink water throughout the day.

Trick: Infuse water with fruit. Infusing water with fruit can be a great way to add flavor and nutrients to water. Some great fruit options include citrus, berries, and cucumbers.

10.6. Tip #5: Get Enough Sleep

Getting enough sleep during pregnancy is essential for maintaining a healthy weight. Lack of sleep can lead to hormonal changes that can increase appetite and lead to weight gain. Additionally, getting enough sleep can help to reduce stress and improve overall health.

Real-life Example: Rachel is a pregnant woman who prioritizes sleep. She goes to bed at the same time every night and sets a consistent sleep schedule. She also avoids caffeine in the evening and creates a relaxing bedtime routine to help her fall asleep.

Trick: Create a sleep-conducive environment. It is important to create a sleep-conducive environment to promote better sleep during pregnancy. Some tips include using blackout curtains, avoiding electronic devices before bed, and keeping the bedroom cool and comfortable.

10.7.   Tools and Anecdote

Tools: Online Resources

There are a variety of online resources available to help women maintain a healthy weight during pregnancy. Some great resources include the American Pregnancy Association and the Centers for Disease Control and Prevention (CDC). These websites provide information on nutrition, exercise, and weight gain during pregnancy.

Anecdote: Jessica's Story

Jessica is a pregnant woman who struggled with weight gain during her first pregnancy. She gained more weight than she wanted to and had trouble losing the weight after giving birth. When she became pregnant with her second child, she was determined to maintain a healthy weight. She consulted with a healthcare provider and created a plan for healthy eating and regular exercise. She also monitored her weight gain and made adjustments to her plan as needed. As a result, she gained a healthy amount of weight during her pregnancy and was able to lose the weight quickly after giving birth.

10.8.   Conclusion

Maintaining a healthy weight during pregnancy is essential for the health of both the mother and the baby. Eating a balanced diet, exercising regularly, monitoring weight gain, drinking plenty of water, and getting enough sleep are all important steps in maintaining a healthy weight during pregnancy. Online resources can also be helpful in providing information and support. By following these tips and tools, women can maintain a healthy weight during pregnancy and improve their overall health and well-being.

11. How to Manage Constipation during Pregnancy

11.1. Introduction

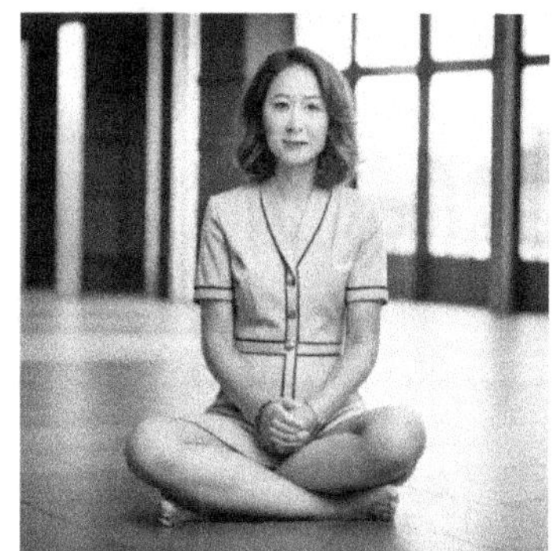

Constipation is a common problem that many pregnant women experience. It is a condition where bowel movements become infrequent, difficult, or painful. It is caused by several factors, including the hormonal changes in the body, an increase in the size of the uterus, and the pressure it puts on the bowels. Constipation can be uncomfortable and frustrating, but there are steps you can take to manage it during pregnancy.

11.2. Tips and Tricks

Here are some tips and tricks that can help you manage constipation during pregnancy:

1. Increase Your Fluid Intake

Drinking plenty of fluids is one of the most effective ways to prevent constipation. Water is the best option, but you can also drink fruit juices, vegetable juices, and herbal teas. You should aim to drink at least eight to ten glasses of fluids per day.

2. Eat High-Fiber Foods

Fiber is essential for maintaining healthy bowel movements. Eating foods high in fiber can help prevent constipation during pregnancy. Some excellent sources of fiber include fruits, vegetables, whole grains, and legumes.

3. Exercise Regularly

Regular exercise can help regulate bowel movements and prevent constipation. Simple activities such as walking, swimming, and yoga can be beneficial during pregnancy. Consult with your healthcare provider before starting any exercise routine during pregnancy.

4. Take Your Prenatal Vitamins

Taking prenatal vitamins can also cause constipation. However, it is essential to continue taking them to ensure that you and your baby receive the necessary nutrients. You can talk to your doctor about switching to a different brand of prenatal vitamins if constipation persists.

5. Use a Squatting Position

Using a squatting position while using the toilet can help relieve constipation. This position allows your colon to straighten out, making it easier to have a bowel movement. You can use a small stool to elevate your feet while sitting on the toilet to achieve this position.

6. Consider Using a Stool Softener

Stool softeners are a type of laxative that can help soften the stool, making it easier to pass. They are safe to use during pregnancy, but you should always consult with your healthcare provider before taking any medication.

7. Avoid Certain Foods

Some foods can worsen constipation during pregnancy. These include processed foods, fried foods, and foods high in fat. Limit your intake of these foods and instead focus on eating a balanced diet that is rich in fiber and nutrients.

8. Manage Your Stress

Stress can contribute to constipation during pregnancy. Finding ways to manage your stress can help alleviate this condition. Some effective stress-management techniques include deep breathing exercises, meditation, and yoga.

9. Get Enough Sleep

Getting enough sleep is crucial during pregnancy. Lack of sleep can cause fatigue and make constipation worse. Try to get at least seven to eight hours of sleep per night and take naps when needed.

10.   Seek Medical Advice

If constipation persists or becomes severe, you should seek medical advice. Your healthcare provider may recommend additional treatments such as suppositories or enemas to help alleviate your symptoms.

11.3.   Real-Life Examples

Constipation during pregnancy can be a frustrating and uncomfortable experience. However, many women have successfully managed this condition with the help of the tips mentioned above. Here are some real-life examples of how women have managed constipation during pregnancy:

Case 1: Sarah was 32 weeks pregnant when she started experiencing constipation. She tried increasing her water intake and eating more fiber-rich foods, but her symptoms persisted. After consulting with her doctor, she started taking a stool softener, which helped alleviate her constipation.

Case 2: Jane was 20 weeks pregnant when she started experiencing constipation. She started practicing yoga and deep breathing exercises, which helped reduce her stress levels and improve her bowel movements.

Case 3: Maria was 28 weeks pregnant when she started experiencing constipation. She tried using a squatting position while using the toilet and increased her fluid intake, but her symptoms persisted. After consulting with her doctor, she started using a stool softener and also added a small amount of prune juice to her diet, which helped regulate her bowel movements.

11.4.   Tricks and Tools

In addition to the tips mentioned above, there are some tricks and tools that can help you manage constipation during pregnancy:

1. **Keep a food diary:** Keeping a food diary can help you identify foods that worsen your constipation. You can use this information to adjust your diet accordingly.

2. **Use a fiber supplement:** If you find it challenging to eat enough fiber-rich foods, you can consider using a fiber supplement. These supplements come in various forms, including powders, pills, and chewable tablets.

3. **Consider acupuncture:** Acupuncture is a form of traditional Chinese medicine that involves the insertion of thin needles into specific points on the body. Some studies have shown that acupuncture can help alleviate constipation during pregnancy.

4. **Use a bidet:** Using a bidet can help clean the anal area without causing irritation, which can be beneficial for women experiencing constipation.

11.5. Conclusion

Constipation is a common problem that many pregnant women experience. However, there are several steps you can take to manage this condition. Increasing your fluid intake, eating high-fiber foods, exercising regularly, and managing your stress levels are just a few of the many tips that can help prevent constipation during pregnancy. If you experience constipation during pregnancy, it is essential to talk to your healthcare provider to ensure that you are using safe and effective treatments. By taking proactive steps to manage your constipation, you can enjoy a more comfortable and healthy pregnancy.

12. How to Deal with Pregnancy-Related Stress

12.1.　Introduction

Pregnancy can be an exciting time, but it can also be a very stressful one. Expectant mothers may experience physical discomfort, hormonal changes, and concerns about the health of their unborn child. These stressors can be 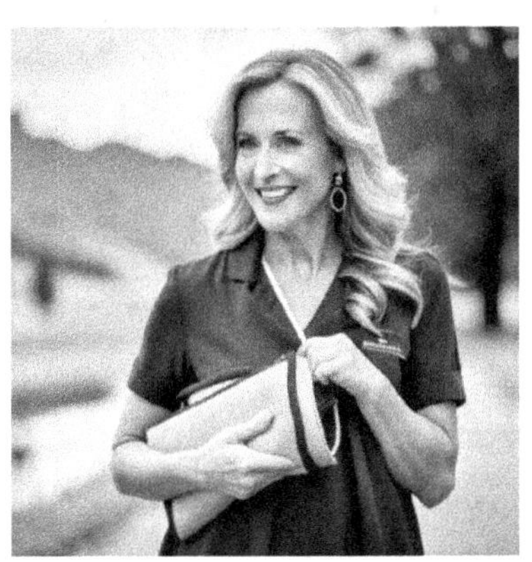 overwhelming, leading to anxiety, depression, and other mental health problems. However, pregnancy-related stress can be managed, and there are a number of strategies that expectant mothers can use to reduce their stress levels and enjoy a healthy and happy pregnancy.

12.2.　Strategies for Dealing with Stress

Here are some tips on how to deal with pregnancy-related stress:

1. Seek support

One of the most important things you can do to deal with pregnancy-related stress is to seek support from family, friends, and healthcare professionals. Talking to someone who understands what you're going through can help to alleviate anxiety and stress. Many women find it helpful to join a pregnancy support group where they can connect with other expectant mothers who are experiencing similar stressors. Alternatively, speaking to a counselor or therapist can provide a safe space to express your concerns and emotions.

2. Practice relaxation techniques

Relaxation techniques such as deep breathing, meditation, and yoga can help to reduce stress levels during pregnancy. These practices can help to calm the mind, reduce physical tension, and promote overall relaxation. There are many resources available online that offer guided meditations and yoga classes specifically designed for pregnant women. Taking a few moments each day to practice relaxation techniques can help to alleviate stress and promote a sense of calm.

3. Stay active

Exercise is an excellent way to manage stress during pregnancy. Not only can it help to reduce stress levels, but it can also improve mood, increase energy levels, and promote overall physical health. It's important to choose activities that are safe and appropriate for your stage of pregnancy. Walking, swimming, and prenatal yoga are all excellent options that can be done throughout pregnancy.

4. Get enough sleep

Sleep is essential for overall health and well-being, but it's especially important during pregnancy. Pregnant women may find it difficult to get comfortable at night, experience frequent urination, and have trouble falling or staying asleep. To promote better sleep, try to establish a regular sleep routine, avoid caffeine and alcohol before bedtime, and create a comfortable sleep environment. This may include investing in a good quality mattress, pillows, and bedding, and ensuring that your room is cool and dark.

5. Manage expectations

Pregnancy can be a time of high expectations, both from ourselves and from others. It's important to manage these expectations and recognize that pregnancy is not always perfect. It's okay to feel overwhelmed, tired, or emotional at times. Try not to compare yourself to others and focus on what is best for you and your baby.

6. Eat well

A healthy diet is essential for both mother and baby during pregnancy. Eating a balanced diet that includes plenty of fruits, vegetables, whole grains, and lean protein can help to reduce stress levels and promote overall health. It's also important to stay hydrated and limit your intake of caffeine and sugar, which can contribute to anxiety and stress.

7. Take breaks

Taking regular breaks throughout the day can help to reduce stress levels and promote a sense of calm. This may include taking a short walk, practicing relaxation techniques, or simply taking a few moments to yourself to rest and recharge. It's important to prioritize self-care during pregnancy and take time for activities that bring you joy and relaxation.

12.3.   Real-life example

Rachel, a 32-year-old mother of two, found pregnancy to be a stressful experience. She felt overwhelmed by the physical discomfort, hormonal changes, and concerns about the health of her unborn child. To manage her stress levels, Rachel sought support from a pregnancy support group and spoke to a counselor about her concerns. She also started practicing prenatal yoga and meditation, which helped to reduce her anxiety and promote relaxation. Additionally, Rachel made sure to prioritize self-care, taking breaks throughout the day to rest and recharge. She also made sure to eat a healthy and balanced diet, which helped to improve her overall mood and energy levels.

12.4.   Tricks and tools

Here are some additional tricks and tools that can help to manage pregnancy-related stress:

1. Keep a journal

Writing down your thoughts and feelings in a journal can be a helpful way to process emotions and reduce stress levels. Taking a few moments each day to reflect on your experiences can provide a sense of clarity and perspective.

2. Practice positive self-talk

Negative self-talk can contribute to feelings of anxiety and stress. Practicing positive self-talk can help to reframe negative thoughts and promote a more positive mindset.

3. Use aromatherapy

Aromatherapy can be a helpful tool for reducing stress levels during pregnancy. Essential oils such as lavender, chamomile, and ylang-ylang can promote relaxation and calm.

4. Seek professional help

If you're experiencing severe or persistent stress and anxiety during pregnancy, it's important to seek professional help. A healthcare professional can provide support and guidance on how to manage your stress levels and promote overall mental health.

12.5.   Conclusion

Pregnancy-related stress can be managed with the right tools and strategies. Seeking support, practicing relaxation techniques, staying active, getting enough sleep, managing expectations, eating well, and taking breaks can all help to reduce stress levels during pregnancy. Remember to prioritize self-care and seek professional help if needed. By taking care of yourself, you can enjoy a healthy and happy pregnancy.

13. How to Recognize and Manage Prenatal Depression

13.1. Introduction

Prenatal depression, also known as antenatal depression, is a form of depression that occurs during pregnancy. It affects about 10-20% of pregnant women, making it one of the most common complications of pregnancy 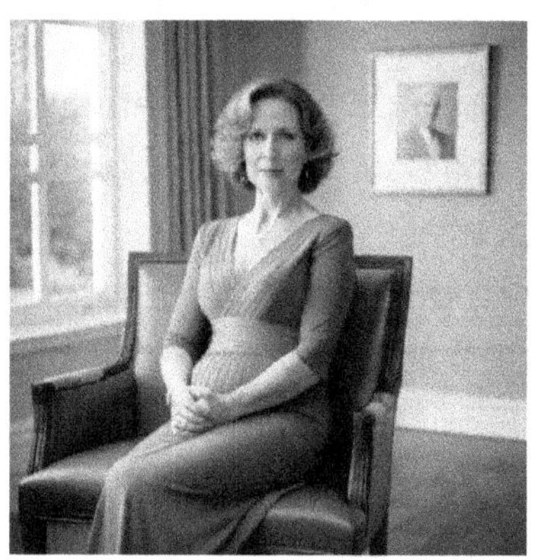 (American College of Obstetricians and Gynecologists. (2018). Depression during pregnancy). Prenatal depression can have a significant impact on the well-being of both the mother and the unborn child. It is essential to recognize and manage prenatal depression to ensure the health and safety of both the mother and the baby.

13.2. Recognizing Prenatal Depression

Recognizing prenatal depression can be challenging because many of its symptoms, such as fatigue, appetite changes, and sleep disturbances, are common during pregnancy. However, if these symptoms persist for more than two weeks and interfere with the woman's ability to function, they may indicate prenatal depression.

Here are some signs and symptoms of prenatal depression to watch for:

1. **Sadness or feelings of hopelessness:** The woman may feel overwhelmed and have a negative outlook on life.

2. **Loss of interest in activities:** She may lose interest in activities that she previously enjoyed, such as hobbies or spending time with friends and family.

3. **Anxiety or irritability:** The woman may feel anxious or irritable and may have trouble relaxing or sleeping.

4. **Changes in appetite:** She may have a decreased or increased appetite and may experience significant weight gain or weight loss.

5. **Sleep disturbances:** She may have trouble sleeping or may sleep more than usual.

6. **Difficulty concentrating:** The woman may have trouble concentrating, remembering things, or making decisions.

7. **Feelings of guilt or worthlessness:** She may feel guilty or worthless and may blame herself for the way she feels.

If you suspect that you or someone you know may be experiencing prenatal depression, it is essential to seek help from a healthcare provider.

13.3.   Managing Prenatal Depression

There are several ways to manage prenatal depression. The treatment approach will depend on the severity of the woman's symptoms and her overall health. Here are some helpful tips to manage prenatal depression:

1. **Talk to your healthcare provider:** If you suspect that you may have prenatal depression, talk to your healthcare provider. They can provide a diagnosis and recommend treatment options based on the severity of your symptoms.

2. **Therapy:** Talk therapy, also known as psychotherapy, can be an effective way to manage prenatal depression. A mental health professional can help the woman identify the underlying causes of her depression and develop coping strategies to manage her symptoms.

3. **Medication:** In some cases, medication may be necessary to manage prenatal depression. Antidepressants can be safe during pregnancy and can help reduce the severity of symptoms.

4. **Support groups:** Joining a support group can be a helpful way to connect with other women who are experiencing similar challenges. Support groups can provide a safe space to share experiences and learn from others.

5. **Self-care:** Practicing self-care can be an effective way to manage prenatal depression. Eating a healthy diet, getting regular exercise, and engaging in activities that promote relaxation and stress reduction can help improve mood and reduce symptoms.

13.4.   Real-Life Examples

Here are some real-life examples of women who have experienced prenatal depression and how they managed their symptoms:

1. **Laura:** Laura had a history of depression and anxiety before becoming pregnant. During her pregnancy, she experienced severe depression and anxiety, which made it difficult for her to function. She sought help from a mental health professional and began talk therapy. With the support of her therapist and family, Laura was able to manage her symptoms and deliver a healthy baby.

2. **Sarah:** Sarah was a first-time mother who had never experienced depression before becoming pregnant. During her second trimester, she began experiencing symptoms of depression, such as fatigue and loss of interest in activities. She talked to her healthcare provider, who recommended that she join a support group. Sarah found the support group to be very helpful in connecting with other women who were going through similar experiences. She also practiced self-care by going for walks and doing prenatal yoga, which helped her manage her symptoms.

3. **Maria:** Maria had a difficult pregnancy and had to be on bed rest for several weeks. This isolation and lack of physical activity contributed to feelings of sadness and hopelessness. She talked to her healthcare provider, who recommended that she try mindfulness meditation. Maria found that practicing mindfulness

helped her manage her symptoms and improve her mood.

13.5.   Tricks and Tools

Here are some tricks and tools that can be helpful in managing prenatal depression:

1. **Journaling:** Writing down thoughts and feelings in a journal can be a helpful way to process emotions and identify triggers for depression.

2. **Meditation and mindfulness:** Practicing meditation and mindfulness can help reduce stress and improve mood.

3. **Exercise:** Regular exercise can help boost mood and improve overall physical and mental health.

4. **Creative expression:** Engaging in creative activities, such as painting or playing music, can be a helpful way to express emotions and reduce stress.

5. **Relaxation techniques:** Practicing relaxation techniques, such as deep breathing or progressive muscle relaxation, can help reduce anxiety and improve sleep.

13.6.   Conclusion

Prenatal depression is a common complication of pregnancy that can have significant impacts on the well-being of both the mother and the unborn child. It is essential to recognize and manage prenatal depression to ensure the health and safety of both. If you suspect that you or someone you know may be experiencing prenatal depression, talk to a healthcare provider. There are several effective treatment options, including therapy, medication, and self-care practices, that can help manage symptoms and improve mood. Remember, seeking help is a sign of strength, and there is no shame in asking for support.

14. How to Practice Self-Care during Pregnancy

14.1. Introduction

Pregnancy is a magical and exciting time in a woman's life, but it can also be physically and emotionally demanding. Taking care of oneself is essential for a healthy pregnancy and an overall positive experience. Self-

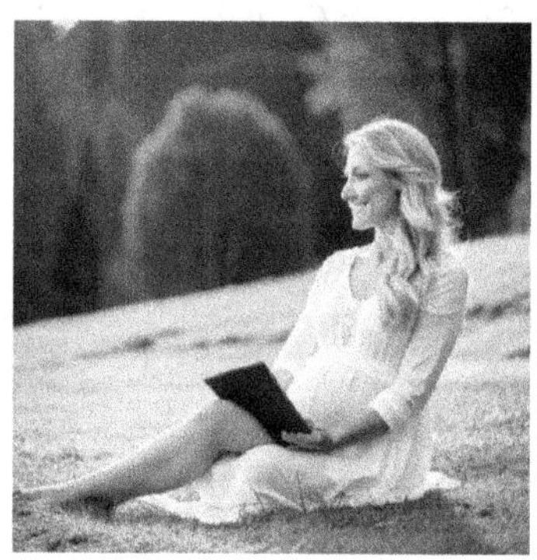

care during pregnancy involves nurturing the body, mind, and soul to support the health of the mother and the growing baby.

14.2. Strategies to Help with Self-Care during Pregnancy

Here are some practical tips and tricks to help you practice self-care during pregnancy.

1. Get Enough Rest:

Getting enough rest is one of the essential things you can do to take care of yourself during pregnancy. Your body is working overtime to grow a new life, so it's essential to get adequate sleep and rest. Try to aim for at least eight hours of sleep each night, and consider taking naps throughout the day. If you have trouble sleeping, try taking a warm bath before bedtime or using relaxation techniques like deep breathing or meditation.

2. Stay Hydrated:

Drinking enough water is crucial for staying healthy during pregnancy. It helps flush out toxins, keeps you hydrated, and supports healthy blood flow to the baby. Aim to drink at least eight glasses of water a day, and consider carrying a reusable water bottle with you everywhere you go to stay hydrated on the go.

3. Eat a Balanced Diet:

Eating a healthy, balanced diet is crucial for both you and your growing baby. Focus on consuming nutrient-dense foods like fruits, vegetables, lean proteins, and whole grains. Avoid processed foods and sugary snacks, which can cause energy crashes and mood swings. If you have trouble getting all the nutrients you need from food, consider taking a prenatal vitamin supplement.

4. Exercise Regularly:

Regular exercise is beneficial for both you and your baby during pregnancy. It can help improve your mood, increase energy levels, and support healthy weight gain. Aim for at least 30 minutes of moderate exercise per day, such as walking, swimming, or prenatal yoga. Always consult with your doctor before starting or changing your exercise routine.

5. Manage Stress:

Stress can be harmful during pregnancy and can lead to a host of physical and emotional issues. It's essential to manage stress levels by practicing relaxation techniques like deep breathing, meditation, or prenatal yoga. Consider making time for activities you enjoy, such as reading, listening to music, or spending time in nature. If you're feeling overwhelmed, don't hesitate to seek support from a mental health professional.

6. Stay Connected:

Staying connected with loved ones is crucial for emotional well-being during pregnancy. Consider joining a prenatal class or support group to connect with other expectant mothers. You can also stay connected with friends and family by sharing updates, photos, and videos throughout your pregnancy.

7. Practice Self-Compassion:

It's essential to practice self-compassion during pregnancy and be kind to yourself. Pregnancy can be physically and emotionally challenging, so it's important to give yourself grace and allow yourself to rest when needed. If you're feeling overwhelmed, try practicing positive affirmations or journaling to help manage your emotions.

8. Take Care of Your Skin:

Your skin can change significantly during pregnancy, so it's essential to take care of it. Use a gentle cleanser and moisturizer to keep your skin hydrated and healthy. You can also try using natural remedies like coconut oil or shea butter to soothe dry skin. Avoid using harsh chemicals or products that can irritate your skin.

9. Prepare for Labor and Delivery:

Preparing for labor and delivery can help ease anxiety and stress during pregnancy. Consider taking a childbirth class or hiring a doula to help you prepare for the big day. You can also practice relaxation techniques like deep breathing, visualization, or hypnobirthing to help manage pain and anxiety during labor.

10.   Plan for Postpartum Care

Planning for postpartum care is an important aspect of self-care during pregnancy. While it's important to focus on a healthy pregnancy and delivery, it's also essential to consider how you'll take care of yourself after the baby is born. Here are some tips for planning for postpartum care:

- *Talk to Your Healthcare Provider:* Your healthcare provider can provide valuable guidance on postpartum care. They can advise you on what to expect during the postpartum period, any warning signs to watch for, and how to care for yourself and your newborn.

- *Create a Postpartum Care Plan:* A postpartum care plan can help you organize your thoughts and plan for your recovery after delivery. Your plan can include information on things like postpartum appointments, breastfeeding support, and any additional support you may need.

- *Arrange for Help:* As mentioned earlier, arranging for help during the postpartum period can be essential for your recovery. Consider hiring a postpartum doula, asking friends and family members to help with household chores or caring for older children, or arranging for meal delivery services.

- **Stock Up on Essentials:** It's a good idea to stock up on essentials before the baby is born. This can include things like sanitary pads, breastfeeding supplies, and healthy snacks.

- **Prioritize Rest and Recovery:** Rest and recovery should continue to be a priority during the postpartum period. Consider arranging for a support system that allows you to take naps and avoid overexerting yourself.

- **Focus on Nutrition:** Just as during pregnancy, nutrition is crucial during the postpartum period. Make sure you're eating nutrient-dense foods and staying hydrated.

- **Attend Postpartum Appointments:** Postpartum appointments are important for monitoring your recovery and ensuring your newborn is healthy. Make sure you attend all scheduled appointments and communicate any concerns with your healthcare provider.

- **Seek Emotional Support:** The postpartum period can be emotionally challenging. Don't hesitate to seek support from friends, family members, or a mental health professional if needed.

- **Be Gentle with Yourself:** It's normal to feel overwhelmed during the postpartum period. Remember to be gentle with yourself and give yourself time to adjust to the demands of motherhood.

- ***Ask for Help:*** Finally, don't hesitate to ask for help when you need it. Taking care of a newborn is a big responsibility, and it's okay to need assistance.

14.3.   Conclusion

Planning for postpartum care is an important aspect of self-care during pregnancy. By talking to your healthcare provider, creating a postpartum care plan, arranging for help, stocking up on essentials, prioritizing rest and recovery, focusing on nutrition, attending postpartum appointments, seeking emotional support, being gentle with yourself, and asking for help when needed, you can help support your physical and emotional well-being during the postpartum period.

15. How to Choose the Right Prenatal Vitamins

15.1.   Introduction

Prenatal vitamins are an essential part of prenatal care for pregnant women. They are designed to provide the extra nutrients and vitamins needed to support a healthy pregnancy and ensure the baby's proper development. But with so many 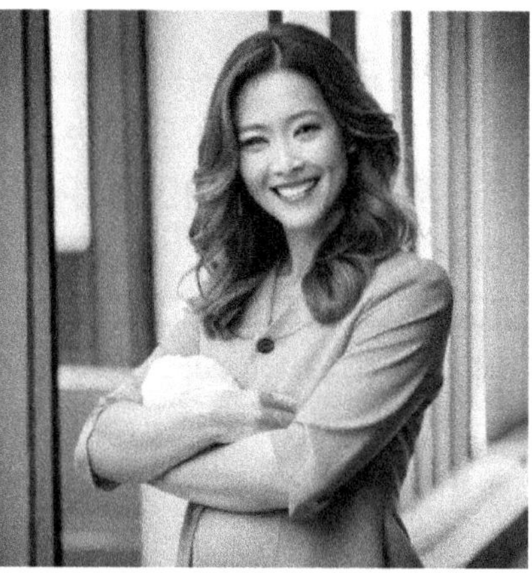 different brands and formulations available, choosing the right prenatal vitamin can be a daunting task. This chapter will guide you through the process of selecting the right prenatal vitamin for you and your baby.

15.2.   Process of Selecting the Right Prenatal Vitamin

1) Understand What You Need

Before you start shopping for prenatal vitamins, it's essential to understand what you need. During pregnancy, your body requires additional nutrients to support your growing baby's development. The most critical nutrients during pregnancy include folic acid, iron, calcium, and vitamin D. Folic acid is essential for preventing birth defects of the baby's brain and spine, known as neural tube defects.

Iron is necessary for the production of red blood cells that carry oxygen to the baby. Calcium is required for the development of strong bones and teeth, and vitamin D helps the body absorb calcium.

2) Consult With Your Doctor

The first step in choosing the right prenatal vitamin is to consult with your doctor. Your doctor will help you determine the appropriate dosage of vitamins and minerals based on your individual needs. Depending on your health history and any underlying medical conditions, your doctor may also recommend additional supplements or a specific brand of prenatal vitamins.

3) Read the Label Carefully

When choosing a prenatal vitamin, it's essential to read the label carefully. Make sure the vitamin contains the essential nutrients needed for a healthy pregnancy. Look for vitamins that contain at least 400-800 mcg of folic acid, 27 mg of iron, 1000 mg of calcium, and 600 IU of vitamin D (March of Dimes. (2021). Prenatal vitamins). It's also important to look at the type of vitamins included in the prenatal vitamin. Some vitamins are easier for the body to absorb and utilize than others. For example, some forms of iron, such as ferrous sulfate, can cause stomach upset and constipation. Consider choosing a prenatal vitamin that contains iron in the form of ferrous bisglycinate, which is gentler on the stomach.

4) Check for Additives and Allergens

When reading the label, it's also important to check for any additives or allergens that may cause an adverse reaction. Some prenatal vitamins may contain artificial colors, flavors, or preservatives that can cause an upset stomach. Look for a vitamin that is free from unnecessary additives. It's also important to check for any allergens. Some prenatal vitamins may contain common allergens such as soy, gluten, or dairy. If you have a food allergy or intolerance, make sure to choose a prenatal vitamin that is free from those allergens.

5) Consider Your Diet

While prenatal vitamins are essential, they should not be a replacement for a healthy diet. A balanced diet rich in fruits, vegetables, whole grains, lean protein, and healthy fats is critical for a healthy pregnancy. Consider choosing a prenatal vitamin that complements your diet and provides any nutrients you may be lacking. For example, if you follow a vegetarian or vegan diet, you may be at risk for iron deficiency. Consider choosing a prenatal vitamin that contains a higher dose of iron or combining your vitamin with an iron-rich food such as spinach or lentils.

6) Look for Third-Party Testing

When choosing a prenatal vitamin, look for products that have been third-party tested. Third-party testing ensures that the product contains the ingredients listed on the label and is free from harmful contaminants. Look for prenatal vitamins that have been certified by organizations such as the United States Pharmacopeia (USP), NSF International, or ConsumerLab.com.

7) Consider Your Budget

Prenatal vitamins can vary in price, with some brands costing more than others. While it's essential to choose a high-quality prenatal vitamin, it's also important to consider your budget when choosing a prenatal vitamin. There are many affordable options on the market that provide all the necessary nutrients. Consider comparing prices and looking for discounts or coupons to save money.

8) Take Your Prenatal Vitamin Consistently

Once you have chosen a prenatal vitamin, it's important to take it consistently. Prenatal vitamins are most effective when taken daily, preferably with a meal. If you have trouble remembering to take your vitamin, try setting a reminder on your phone or keeping them in a visible location.

15.3.   Real-Life Examples

Choosing the right prenatal vitamin can make a significant difference in your pregnancy and your baby's development. For example, when Samantha, a first-time mom, found out she was pregnant, she was overwhelmed with the number of prenatal vitamins available. After consulting with her doctor and doing research, she chose a prenatal vitamin that contained the necessary nutrients and was free from additives and allergens. She took her vitamin daily and had a healthy pregnancy and delivery.

15.4.   Tricks and Tools

Here are some additional tricks and tools to help you choose the right prenatal vitamin:

- Consider choosing a prenatal vitamin that contains DHA, an omega-3 fatty acid that supports the baby's brain and eye development.

- If you experience nausea or morning sickness, consider taking your prenatal vitamin before bed or with a small snack.

- Look for prenatal vitamins that come in easy-to-swallow capsules or gummies if you have trouble with large pills.

- If you have trouble swallowing pills altogether, consider a prenatal vitamin that comes in a liquid form.

15.5.   Conclusion

Choosing the right prenatal vitamin is an essential part of a healthy pregnancy. It's important to consult with your doctor, read the label carefully, consider your diet, and look for third-party testing when selecting a prenatal vitamin. Taking your vitamin consistently and considering your budget can also make a significant difference. With these tips, tricks, and tools, you can choose the right prenatal vitamin for you and your baby and have a healthy pregnancy and delivery.

16. How to Prepare For Childbirth and Labor

16.1.   Introduction

Childbirth and labor can be a daunting experience for any expectant mother. However, proper preparation can help alleviate some of the anxiety and stress associated with childbirth. This chapter will 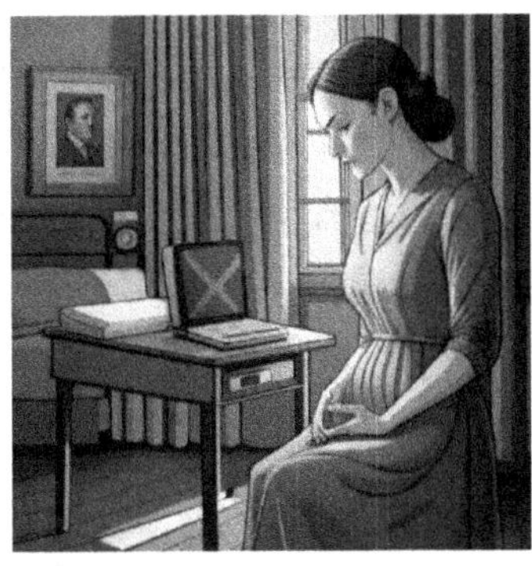 discuss some tips, tricks, and tools that can help you prepare for childbirth and labor.

16.2.   Preparing for Childbirth and Labor

1. **Attend Prenatal Classes:** Prenatal classes are an excellent way to learn about childbirth, labor, and the postpartum period. These classes are typically offered by hospitals, childbirth educators, and doulas. Prenatal classes provide expectant mothers with valuable information on breathing and relaxation techniques, pain management options, and labor positions. Prenatal classes can also help you connect with other expectant mothers, which can be a great source of support during your pregnancy and beyond.

2. **Exercise:** Exercise is essential during pregnancy as it can help prepare your body for labor and childbirth. Exercise can also help improve your mood and reduce

stress and anxiety. However, it's important to consult with your healthcare provider before starting any exercise program during pregnancy. Low-impact exercises like walking, swimming, and prenatal yoga are generally safe for most pregnant women.

3. **Prepare for Labor:** Labor can be unpredictable, and it's essential to be prepared for all eventualities. Pack a hospital bag with all the essentials you will need for your stay, including comfortable clothes, toiletries, and items for your baby. Make sure to discuss your birth plan with your healthcare provider and your birth partner, so everyone is on the same page. Consider hiring a doula or a birth photographer to help support you during labor and capture those precious moments.

4. **Create a Relaxing Environment:** Labor can be intense, and creating a relaxing environment can help you manage the pain and stress associated with childbirth. Consider using aromatherapy, playing relaxing music, or bringing comforting items from home, like a favorite pillow or blanket. You can also consider creating a birth playlist with songs that calm you and help you stay focused during labor.

5. **Practice Breathing Techniques:** Breathing techniques can help you stay calm and focused during labor. Practicing different breathing techniques can help you find the right one that works best for you. Some popular breathing techniques include deep breathing, slow breathing, and patterned breathing. Consider attending prenatal classes or practicing with

your birth partner to find the best breathing technique for you.

6. **Consider Pain Management Options:** Pain is a normal part of labor, but there are several pain management options available to help you manage the discomfort. Some pain management options include epidurals, nitrous oxide, and other medication options. Discuss these options with your healthcare provider and make an informed decision about what pain management option is best for you.

7. **Stay Hydrated:** Staying hydrated during labor is essential to ensure you have enough energy and to prevent dehydration. Drink plenty of water, and consider packing drinks like coconut water or sports drinks that can help replenish electrolytes lost during labor.

8. **Practice Labor Positions:** Labor positions can help you manage the pain and discomfort associated with childbirth. Experiment with different positions, such as standing, squatting, or using a birthing ball, to find what works best for you. Labor positions can also help facilitate the birth process and reduce the risk of complications.

9. **Keep an Open Mind:** Labor and childbirth can be unpredictable, and it's important to keep an open mind and be flexible with your birth plan. Remember that the ultimate goal is to deliver a healthy baby, and sometimes unexpected things happen. Be prepared to

adjust your plans and trust your healthcare provider to make the best decisions for you and your baby.

10.   **Have a Support System:** Having a strong support system during labor and childbirth can make all the difference. Consider having your partner, family member, or friend with you during labor, or hire a doula to provide additional support. A doula is a trained professional who can provide emotional, physical, and informational support during labor and childbirth. Doulas can help you navigate the labor process, provide comfort measures, and advocate for your wishes and preferences.

11.   **Practice Relaxation Techniques:** Relaxation techniques, such as visualization, meditation, and progressive muscle relaxation, can help you stay calm and focused during labor. Practicing relaxation techniques during pregnancy can help you build the skills you need to manage pain and stress during labor. Consider attending prenatal classes or practicing with your birth partner to learn different relaxation techniques.

12.   **Get Plenty of Rest:** Rest is essential during pregnancy and especially important during labor. Make sure to get plenty of rest in the weeks leading up to your due date, and try to conserve your energy during labor. Consider taking naps or breaks during early labor to help you conserve your energy for the later stages of labor.

13. **Eat Nutritious Foods:** Eating nutritious foods during pregnancy and labor is essential to ensure you have the energy and nutrients you need for the birthing process. Consider packing snacks like nuts, fruits, and granola bars to eat during labor. Eating small, frequent meals can also help keep your energy levels up during the birthing process.

14. **Educate Yourself:** Educating yourself about childbirth and labor can help you feel more prepared and confident. Read books, attend prenatal classes, and talk to your healthcare provider to learn more about the birthing process. Knowing what to expect can help you feel more in control and empowered during labor.

16.3. Conclusion

Preparing for childbirth and labor can help alleviate some of the anxiety and stress associated with the birthing process. Attending prenatal classes, exercising, preparing for labor, creating a relaxing environment, practicing breathing and relaxation techniques, considering pain management options, staying hydrated, practicing labor positions, keeping an open mind, having a support system, practicing relaxation techniques, getting plenty of rest, eating nutritious foods, and educating yourself can all help you prepare for childbirth and labor. Remember that every birth experience is unique, and it's essential to trust your healthcare provider and be flexible with your birth plan. With proper preparation and support, you can have a positive and empowering birth experience.

17. How to Create a Birth Plan

17.1. Introduction

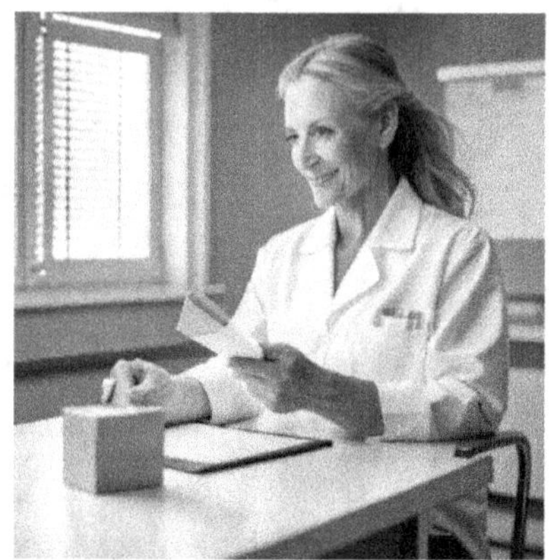

A birth plan is a written document that outlines your preferences for labor, delivery, and postpartum care. It's an essential tool for communicating your wishes with your healthcare provider, partner, and anyone else involved in your birth experience. The birth plan helps you take control of your birth experience and ensures that you and your baby receive the care you want and need. Creating a birth plan may seem like a daunting task, especially if you are a first-time parent. However, with a little preparation and research, you can create a birth plan that reflects your values, priorities, and preferences. Here are some tips, tricks, and tools to help you create a birth plan that works for you.

17.2. Strategies for Creating a Birth Plan that Works

1. Research your options

Before creating a birth plan, it's essential to educate yourself on the different options available for labor, delivery, and postpartum care. Talk to your healthcare provider, read books, attend childbirth classes, and seek advice from other parents. Familiarize yourself with the benefits and risks of different interventions and procedures, so you can make informed decisions about your birth preferences.

2. Decide on your birth team

Your birth team consists of your healthcare provider, partner, doula, and anyone else who will be present during your birth. Consider your relationship with your healthcare provider and their philosophy on birth. Decide whether you want to hire a doula or other support person to advocate for you during labor and delivery. Discuss your birth plan with your partner and make sure they are on board with your preferences.

3. Prioritize your preferences

When creating your birth plan, it's essential to prioritize your preferences. Rank your preferences in order of importance, so you can communicate your top priorities to your healthcare provider. For example, you may prioritize having a vaginal birth without pain medication, but you are willing to consider an epidural if necessary. Be flexible and open to changes, as birth is unpredictable, and your preferences may change during labor.

4. Be specific and clear

When writing your birth plan, be specific and clear about your preferences. Use clear, concise language and avoid medical jargon. Include details about your preferences for pain management, labor positions, monitoring, pushing, and delivery. Specify whether you want to have a vaginal birth or a cesarean delivery, and if you have a preference for a specific type of anesthesia. Include details about your preferences for skin-to-skin contact, breastfeeding, and postpartum care.

5. Include contingency plans

Birth is unpredictable, and it's important to include contingency plans in your birth plan. Consider different scenarios that may arise, such as fetal distress, a prolonged labor, or the need for a cesarean delivery. Include your preferences for these situations, so your healthcare provider knows what you want. For example, you may want to specify that you want to avoid a cesarean delivery unless it's medically necessary.

6. Use templates and examples

There are many templates and examples available online that can help you create your birth plan. Use these resources as a starting point, and customize them to reflect your preferences. Remember, your birth plan should be unique to you and your birth experience, so don't be afraid to make changes and revisions as necessary.

7. Review and revise

Once you have created your birth plan, review it with your healthcare provider and birth team. Make sure everyone is on the same page and understands your preferences. Review and revise your birth plan as necessary, especially as your due date approaches. Remember, your birth plan is a flexible document that can change as your needs and preferences change.

17.3.   Real-life examples

Here are some real-life examples of birth plans that reflect different preferences and priorities:

Example 1:

NAME:	**SARAH JOHNSON**
DUE DATE:	May 15, 2023
BIRTH PREFERENCES:	<ul><li>Vaginal birth without pain medication</li><li>Labor and delivery in a birthing center</li><li>Use of a birthing ball, massage, and breathing techniques for pain management</li><li>Freedom to move and change positions during labor</li><li>Limited vaginal exams and interventions</li><li>Delayed cord clamping and immediate skin-to-skin contact with baby</li><li>Exclusive breastfeeding and rooming-in</li><li>Avoidance of routine procedures such as eye ointment and vitamin K shot</li></ul>

Example 2:

Name:	**John and Emily Smith**
Due Date:	July 1, 2023
Birth Preferences:	• Vaginal birth with epidural anesthesia • Labor and delivery in a hospital with access to a neonatal intensive care unit (NICU) • Use of a birthing ball, massage, and breathing techniques for pain management • Frequent monitoring of baby's heart rate • Freedom to move and change positions during labor • Limited vaginal exams and interventions • Delayed cord clamping and immediate skin-to-skin contact with baby • Exclusive breastfeeding and rooming-in • Openness to cesarean delivery if medically necessary

Example 3:

Name:	**Maria Rodriguez**
Due Date:	September 15, 2023
Birth Preferences:	• Vaginal birth with limited interventions • Labor and delivery in a hospital with access to pain medication if needed • Use of a birthing ball, massage, and breathing techniques for pain management • Freedom to move and change positions during labor • Limited vaginal exams and interventions • Delayed cord clamping and immediate skin-to-skin contact with baby • Exclusive breastfeeding and rooming-in • Avoidance of routine procedures such as episiotomy, forceps, and vacuum extraction

17.4. Tricks and Tools

Here are some tricks and tools that can help you create a birth plan that works for you:

- Use a birth plan worksheet or template to organize your preferences.

- Consider hiring a doula or other support person to advocate for you during labor and delivery.

- Attend childbirth classes and read books to educate yourself on your options.

- Discuss your birth plan with your healthcare provider and birth team.

- Consider using a birth plan app or website to create and customize your birth plan.

- Be flexible and open to changes, as birth is unpredictable.

- Review and revise your birth plan as necessary, especially as your due date approaches.

17.5. Conclusion

Creating a birth plan can help you take control of your birth experience and ensure that you and your baby receive the care you want and need. By researching your options, prioritizing your preferences, being specific and clear, including contingency plans, using templates and examples, and reviewing and revising your birth plan, you can create a document that reflects your values and priorities. Remember, your birth plan is a flexible document that can change as your needs and preferences change. With a little preparation and research, you can create a birth plan that works for you and your family.

18. How to Prepare For a C-Section

18.1.   Introduction

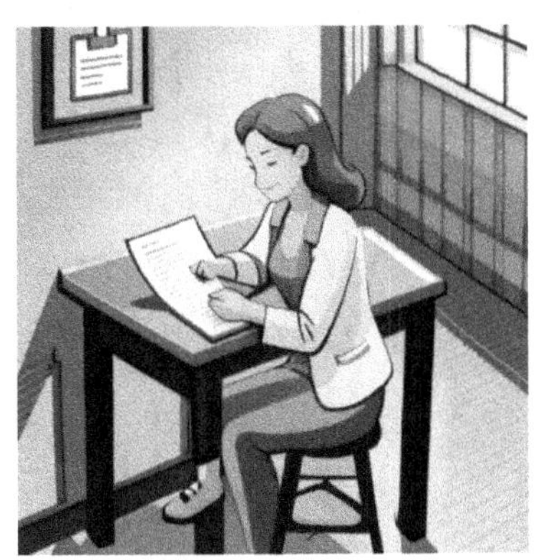

A Cesarean delivery, commonly known as a C-section, is a surgical procedure that involves delivering a baby through an incision made in the mother's abdomen and uterus. While most women hope for a natural birth, sometimes a C-section may be necessary due to certain medical conditions or complications during pregnancy. If you have been advised to have a C-section, it is important to know what to expect and how to prepare. This chapter will discuss some helpful tips, real-life examples, anecdotes, tricks, and tools that readers can use to prepare for a C-section.

18.2.   Preparing for a C-Section

1. Know what to expect

Before you prepare for a C-section, it is important to understand what the procedure involves. A C-section is a surgical procedure that involves making a small incision in your abdomen and uterus to deliver the baby. You will be given anesthesia to numb the lower part of your body, and you will be awake during the procedure. The procedure itself usually takes about 30 minutes, but you will need to stay in the hospital for a few days to recover.

2. Discuss your concerns with your healthcare provider

It is important to discuss your concerns about the C-section with your healthcare provider. They can provide you with more information about the procedure, answer your questions, and address any fears or concerns you may have. They may also provide you with resources, such as books or websites that can help you prepare for the C-section.

3. Pack a hospital bag

Just like with a natural birth, it is important to pack a hospital bag for a C-section. You will need comfortable clothes to wear during your hospital stay, such as loose-fitting pants and tops that are easy to breastfeed in. You should also bring a nursing bra, breast pads, and comfortable shoes. Other items to pack include toiletries, such as toothbrush and toothpaste, shampoo and conditioner, and body lotion. Don't forget to bring items that will help you pass the time, such as books, magazines, and music.

4. Arrange for help at home

After a C-section, you will need time to recover, and it may be difficult to perform everyday tasks, such as cooking, cleaning, and taking care of your newborn. It is important to arrange for help at home, such as a family member or friend who can assist you with these tasks. If you do not have anyone who can help you, consider hiring a postpartum doula or a home health aide.

5. Rest as much as possible before the C-section

It is important to rest as much as possible before the C-section. This will help you to conserve your energy and prepare for the surgery. Get plenty of sleep, eat healthy foods, and avoid strenuous activities. Try to stay relaxed and calm, as stress and anxiety can make the recovery process more difficult.

6. Understand the risks and benefits of the procedure

Like with any medical procedure, a C-section comes with risks and benefits. It is important to understand these risks and benefits so that you can make an informed decision about the procedure. Some benefits of a C-section include a lower risk of certain complications, such as pelvic floor damage and incontinence. However, there are also risks, such as infection, bleeding, and blood clots. Your healthcare provider can provide you with more information about the risks and benefits of the procedure.

7. Prepare for the recovery process

The recovery process after a C-section can be challenging, so it is important to prepare for it. You will need to take it easy for a few weeks, avoid strenuous activities, and get plenty of rest. You may experience pain, discomfort, and fatigue during the recovery process. It is important to follow your healthcare provider's instructions for pain management and to take any prescribed medications as directed. You may also want to invest in some postpartum recovery essentials, such as a nursing pillow, a belly binder, and comfortable nursing bras.

8. Learn about breastfeeding after a C-section

Breastfeeding after a C-section can be a bit more challenging than with a natural birth, but it is still possible. It may take a bit longer for your milk to come in, and you may need to use certain positions and techniques to help your baby latch on properly. Consider taking a breastfeeding class before the birth, and ask your healthcare provider or a lactation consultant for advice and support.

9. Practice relaxation techniques

Practicing relaxation techniques can help you stay calm and reduce stress and anxiety before and after the C-section. Consider practicing deep breathing, meditation, yoga, or other relaxation techniques that work for you. You may also want to try visualization exercises, such as imagining yourself in a peaceful and calming environment.

10.   Stay positive and focus on the end goal

A C-section may not be what you had hoped for, but it is important to stay positive and focus on the end goal – a healthy baby and a healthy mom. Remember that the C-section is just one part of the journey, and that there are many joys and challenges to come with being a new parent. Focus on the positives, such as the opportunity to bond with your baby, and don't be afraid to ask for help and support when you need it.

18.3.   Real-life examples

Many women have shared their experiences and tips for preparing for a C-section. Here are a few examples:

- "I was really scared about the C-section, but my doctor and nurses were amazing. They talked me through every step of the procedure and made me feel comfortable and safe. I also found that packing a hospital bag with all my essentials, including some comforting items from home, helped me feel more at ease during my hospital stay." - Sarah, mother of one

- "Breastfeeding after my C-section was a bit of a challenge, but I found that using a nursing pillow and different positions helped a lot. I also took advantage of the lactation consultant at the hospital, who provided me with lots of advice and support." - Jessica, mother of two

- "After my C-section, I made sure to rest as much as possible and accept help from family and friends. I also invested in a good belly binder, which helped with the pain and discomfort during the recovery process." - Amanda, mother of three

18.4.   Tricks and tools

Here are some tricks and tools that can help you prepare for a C-section:

- Use a pregnancy app or website to track your symptoms, appointments, and progress during pregnancy.
- Practice relaxation techniques, such as deep breathing, meditation, or yoga, to help you stay calm and reduce stress and anxiety.
- Invest in postpartum recovery essentials, such as a nursing pillow, a belly binder, and comfortable nursing bras.

- Attend a breastfeeding class before the birth, and ask your healthcare provider or a lactation consultant for advice and support.
- Pack a hospital bag with all your essentials, including comfortable clothes, toiletries, and items that will help you pass the time.
- Arrange for help at home, such as a family member or friend who can assist you with everyday tasks.
- Follow your healthcare provider's instructions for pain management and take any prescribed medications as directed.

18.5.   Conclusion

Preparing for a C-section can be a bit intimidating, but with the right information, support, and tools, you can make the process smoother and more manageable. Remember to talk to your healthcare provider about any concerns or questions you may have, pack a hospital bag with all your essentials, and arrange for help at home. Practice relaxation techniques, invest in postpartum recovery essentials, and stay positive and focused on the end goal – a healthy baby and a healthy mom. While a C-section may not be what you had hoped for, it can be a lifesaving procedure for you and your baby. By taking the time to prepare and educate yourself, you can ensure that you are ready for whatever comes your way. Remember to focus on the positives, stay calm, and ask for help when you need it. With these tips and tools, you can prepare for a C-section and feel confident and empowered as you welcome your new little one into the world.

19. How to Breastfeed Your Newborn Baby

19.1.　　Introduction

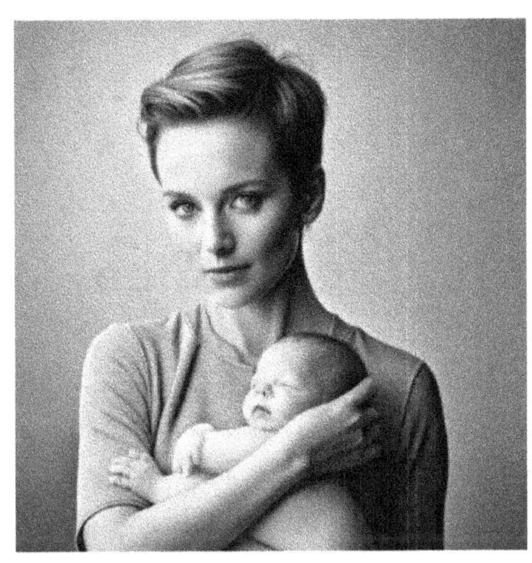

Breastfeeding is a wonderful way to bond with your newborn baby while providing the best possible nutrition for their growth and development. However, it can also be challenging for new mothers who may struggle with latching, milk production, and finding a comfortable position. This chapter will provide helpful tips, real-life examples, anecdotes, tricks, and tools for how to breastfeed your newborn baby.

19.2.　　Preparing to Breastfeed

Before your baby arrives, it is important to prepare yourself for breastfeeding. This includes understanding the benefits of breastfeeding, seeking support from healthcare professionals, and learning about proper positioning and latching techniques. One of the most important benefits of breastfeeding is that it provides all the nutrients your baby needs for the first six months of life. Breast milk contains antibodies that can protect your baby from infections and illnesses, and it can also help reduce the risk of sudden infant death syndrome (SIDS) and childhood obesity.

Additionally, breastfeeding can help you bond with your baby and may even help reduce your risk of breast and ovarian cancer. To ensure that you have the support you need, it is a good idea to talk to your healthcare provider or a lactation consultant before your baby is born. They can answer your questions and provide you with resources such as breastfeeding classes, support groups, and information on breastfeeding-friendly hospitals and clinics.

19.3.   Positioning and Latching

When it comes to breastfeeding, finding a comfortable position for both you and your baby is key. There are several positions you can try, including the cradle hold, football hold, and side-lying position. Experiment with different positions until you find one that feels comfortable and allows your baby to latch onto your breast properly. Latching is the process of attaching your baby to your breast so they can feed. To ensure a good latch, make sure your baby is positioned correctly and that their mouth is wide open. When your baby latches correctly, their lips should be turned outward, and they should have a large portion of your areola (the dark area around your nipple) in their mouth. If you are struggling with latching, try expressing a small amount of milk onto your nipple to encourage your baby to open their mouth wider. You can also gently stroke your baby's cheek to stimulate them to turn their head towards your breast.

19.4.   Milk Production

Breast milk production works on a supply and demand basis, which means that the more your baby feeds, the more milk your body will produce. It is important to feed your baby whenever they are hungry, which is typically every 2-3 hours in the first few weeks of life. If you are having trouble producing enough milk, there are several things you can try. First, make sure you are drinking enough fluids and eating a healthy, balanced diet. You can also try pumping after feedings to help increase your milk production. Additionally, some women find that certain herbs such as fenugreek or blessed thistle can help increase milk production, but it is important to talk to your healthcare provider before trying any supplements.

19.5.   Common Challenges

Breastfeeding can be challenging, and many new mothers face issues such as sore nipples, engorgement, and mastitis. If you experience any of these issues, it is important to seek help from a healthcare professional. Sore nipples are a common problem in the early weeks of breastfeeding. To reduce discomfort, make sure your baby is latching correctly and try using lanolin cream or coconut oil to soothe your nipples. You can also try expressing a small amount of milk onto your nipples and letting it air dry.

Engorgement occurs when your breasts become overly full with milk, which can cause discomfort and make it difficult for your baby to latch. To alleviate engorgement, try applying warm compresses to your breasts before feeding and cold compresses after feeding. You can also try expressing a small amount of milk before feedings to soften the areola and make it easier for your baby to latch. Mastitis is an infection of the breast tissue that can cause flu-like symptoms, fever, and redness or pain in the breast. If you suspect you have mastitis, it is important to seek medical attention right away. Your healthcare provider may prescribe antibiotics to treat the infection, and they may also recommend using warm compresses and getting plenty of rest.

19.6.   Tips for Successful Breastfeeding

Here are some additional tips to help make breastfeeding a success for you and your baby:

- **Be patient:** Breastfeeding can take time to master, so be patient with yourself and your baby as you learn together.

- **Get comfortable:** Make sure you are in a comfortable position with plenty of support for your back and arms.

- **Take breaks:** Breastfeeding can be tiring, so make sure to take breaks and rest as needed.

- **Stay hydrated:** Drinking plenty of fluids can help keep your milk production up.

- **Seek support:** Don't be afraid to reach out to your healthcare provider, a lactation consultant, or a support group for help and guidance.

- **Take care of yourself:** Remember to take care of your own physical and emotional needs so that you can be the best possible caregiver for your baby.

19.7.   Conclusion

Breastfeeding is a wonderful way to bond with your newborn baby while providing them with the best possible nutrition. While it can be challenging at times, with the right preparation, positioning, and support, it can also be a rewarding and fulfilling experience. Remember to be patient with yourself and your baby, and don't hesitate to seek help if you encounter any challenges along the way. With time, practice, and support, you can successfully breastfeed your newborn and enjoy all the benefits that come with it.

20. How to Manage Postpartum Depression

20.1.　　　Introduction

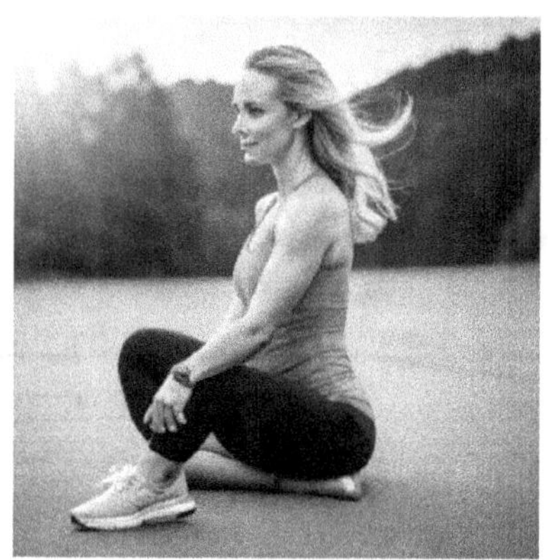

Postpartum depression (PPD) is a common mood disorder that affects many new mothers. It is estimated that up to 20% of women experience PPD after giving birth (American Psychological Association). The symptoms of PPD can range from mild to severe and can include feelings of sadness, anxiety, irritability, and difficulty bonding with the baby. PPD is a serious condition that requires proper management and treatment. This chapter will discuss how to manage postpartum depression and provide helpful tips and tools for new mothers.

20.2.　　　Tip #1: Seek Help from a Mental Health Professional

If you suspect that you may have PPD, it is important to seek help from a mental health professional. A mental health professional can provide you with a proper diagnosis and recommend treatment options. Treatment for PPD can include talk therapy, medication, or a combination of both. Your mental health professional can work with you to develop a treatment plan that is tailored to your specific needs.

Real-Life Example:

After giving birth to her second child, Maria began to feel overwhelmed, anxious, and sad. She found it difficult to bond with her baby and often felt like a failure as a mother. Maria's husband encouraged her to seek help from a mental health professional. After a few sessions with a therapist, Maria was diagnosed with PPD and started on medication. With the help of her therapist and medication, Maria was able to manage her symptoms and develop a stronger bond with her baby.

20.3.   Tip #2: Practice Self-Care

Self-care is essential for managing PPD. As a new mother, it can be challenging to find time for yourself, but it is important to prioritize self-care. This can include things like taking a relaxing bath, reading a book, or going for a walk. It is important to remember that taking care of yourself is not selfish, it is necessary for your mental health.

Real-Life Example:

Emma, a new mother, found it challenging to find time for self-care. She felt guilty leaving her baby to take a break, but soon realized that taking care of herself was essential for her mental health. Emma started taking short walks during her baby's nap time and found that it helped her clear her mind and feel more relaxed.

20.4.　　Tip #3: Build a Support System

Building a support system is essential for managing PPD. This can include family members, friends, or a support group. It is important to have people in your life who can provide emotional support and help with practical tasks, like cooking or cleaning. Having a support system can help reduce feelings of isolation and provide a sense of community.

Real-Life Example:

When Sarah gave birth to her first child, she felt overwhelmed and alone. She found it challenging to manage her PPD symptoms while taking care of her baby. Sarah reached out to a support group for new mothers and found a community of women who were going through similar experiences. Through the support group, Sarah was able to find emotional support and practical advice for managing PPD.

20.5.　　Tip #4: Get Enough Sleep

Sleep is essential for managing PPD. Lack of sleep can exacerbate symptoms of depression and anxiety. It is important to prioritize sleep and create a sleep routine that works for you. This can include things like avoiding caffeine before bed, creating a relaxing bedtime routine, and taking naps when possible.

Real-Life Example:

Jen, a new mother, found it challenging to get enough sleep with a newborn baby. She felt exhausted and overwhelmed, which made it difficult to manage her PPD symptoms. Jen's husband started taking over some of the nighttime feedings, which allowed Jen to get a few hours of uninterrupted sleep. With the help of her husband, Jen was able to prioritize sleep and manage her PPD symptoms more effectively.

20.6.　　　Tip #5: Practice Mindfulness

Mindfulness is a powerful tool for managing PPD. Mindfulness involves being present in the moment and focusing on your thoughts and emotions without judgment. It can help reduce feelings of anxiety and depression and promote feelings of calm and relaxation. Mindfulness can be practiced through meditation, deep breathing exercises, or simply taking a few minutes to focus on your breath.

Real-Life Example:

After giving birth to her third child, Rachel experienced severe PPD symptoms. She found it challenging to manage her emotions and felt overwhelmed most of the time. Rachel started practicing mindfulness meditation for a few minutes each day. She found that focusing on her breath helped her feel more centered and calm. Over time, Rachel's PPD symptoms began to improve, and she was able to manage her emotions more effectively.

20.7.　　　Tip #6: Communicate with Your Partner

Communicating with your partner is essential for managing PPD. Your partner can provide emotional support and help with practical tasks. It is important to be open and honest about your feelings and let your partner know how they can best support you.

Real-Life Example:

After giving birth to her second child, Laura experienced severe PPD symptoms. She found it difficult to communicate her feelings to her husband and often felt like a burden. Laura's husband encouraged her to be open and honest about her emotions and let him know how he could support her. With her husband's support, Laura was able to manage her PPD symptoms and develop a stronger bond with her baby.

20.8.   Conclusion

Managing postpartum depression is essential for new mothers. Seeking help from a mental health professional, practicing self-care, building a support system, getting enough sleep, practicing mindfulness, and communicating with your partner are all effective strategies for managing PPD. It is important to remember that PPD is a common condition and that there is no shame in seeking help. With proper treatment and support, new mothers can overcome PPD and enjoy the joys of motherhood.

21. Conclusion

21.1.　Introduction

Pregnancy is a special time in a woman's life. It's a time when your body is undergoing significant changes and the growth of a new life is taking place inside you. The journey of pregnancy can be both exciting and challenging, and it's 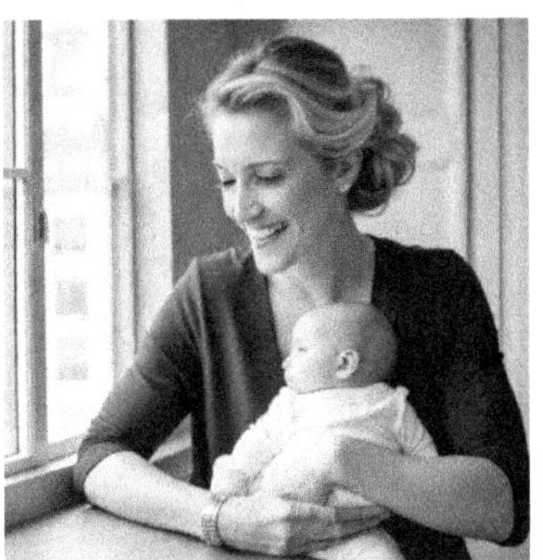 important to take care of yourself and your baby. This comprehensive guide has covered everything you need to know about having a healthy pregnancy, from what to eat to how to manage stress.

21.2.　Healthy Eating

A healthy diet is crucial during pregnancy as it provides the nutrients necessary for your baby's growth and development. A well-balanced diet should include protein, carbohydrates, healthy fats, vitamins, and minerals. Here are some tips for healthy eating during pregnancy:

1. **Eat a variety of foods** - Include a variety of fruits, vegetables, whole grains, lean protein, and healthy fats in your diet.

2. **Stay hydrated** - Drink plenty of water throughout the day to prevent dehydration.

3. **Avoid certain foods** - Avoid raw or undercooked meat, fish with high mercury levels, and unpasteurized dairy products as they can increase the risk of foodborne illness.

4. **Take a prenatal vitamin** - Prenatal vitamins help fill the nutritional gaps in your diet and provide essential nutrients like folic acid, iron, and calcium.

5. **Limit caffeine** - Caffeine intake should be limited to 200 milligrams per day, which is about one 12-ounce cup of coffee.

Real-Life Example: "During my pregnancy, I made sure to eat a variety of foods to ensure I was getting all the necessary nutrients. I also drank plenty of water and avoided sushi, deli meat, and other foods that could potentially harm my baby."

21.3.   Exercise and Physical Activity

Staying active during pregnancy is important for both you and your baby. Regular exercise can help you maintain a healthy weight, reduce stress, and improve your mood. However, it's important to talk to your healthcare provider before starting any exercise program. Here are some tips for exercising during pregnancy:

1. **Choose low-impact activities** - Activities like walking, swimming, and prenatal yoga are low-impact and safe for most pregnant women.

2. **Listen to your body** - If an exercise feels uncomfortable or causes pain, stop immediately.

3. **Stay cool** - Avoid exercising in hot and humid conditions as it can increase your risk of dehydration and overheating.

4. **Wear comfortable clothing** - Choose loose-fitting and breathable clothing that allows for movement and helps regulate body temperature.

5. **Stay hydrated** - Drink plenty of water before, during, and after exercise to prevent dehydration.

Real-Life Example: "I continued my regular workout routine during my pregnancy, but I made some modifications. I switched to low-impact activities like walking and yoga and made sure to stay cool and hydrated during my workouts."

21.4. Managing Stress

Pregnancy can be stressful, and it's important to manage stress to avoid negative effects on you and your baby's health. Here are some tips for managing stress during pregnancy:

1. **Practice relaxation techniques** - Techniques like deep breathing, meditation, and prenatal yoga can help reduce stress.

2. **Get plenty of rest** - Aim for 7-9 hours of sleep per night to help reduce stress and improve overall health.

3. **Stay organized** - Create a to-do list and prioritize tasks to avoid feeling overwhelmed.

4. **Seek support** - Talk to friends, family, or a healthcare provider if you're feeling stressed or anxious.

5. **Take breaks** - Schedule regular breaks throughout the day to rest and recharge.

Real-Life Example: "I found prenatal yoga and meditation to be helpful in managing my stress during pregnancy. I also made sure to get plenty of rest and took breaks throughout the day to avoid feeling overwhelmed."

21.5. Preparing for Labor and Delivery

Preparing for labor and delivery can help you feel more confident and in control during the birthing process. Here are some tips for preparing for labor and delivery:

1. **Take childbirth classes** - Childbirth classes can help you learn about the stages of labor, pain management techniques, and what to expect during delivery.

2. **Create a birth plan** - A birth plan outlines your preferences for labor, delivery, and postpartum care.

3. **Pack a hospital bag** - Pack a bag with essentials like clothes, toiletries, and a camera.

4. **Consider pain management options** - Talk to your healthcare provider about pain management options like epidurals, breathing techniques, or other pain relief methods.

5. **Choose a support person** - Consider who you want to be with you during labor and delivery, whether it's your partner, family member, or doula.

Real-Life Example: "I took a childbirth class to prepare for labor and delivery and created a birth plan that included my preferences for pain management and postpartum care. I also packed a hospital bag and had my partner with me during the birthing process."

21.6.   Postpartum Care

After your baby is born, postpartum care is essential for your physical and emotional recovery. Here are some tips for postpartum care:

1. **Rest and recover** - Take time to rest and recover after childbirth, and don't feel guilty about asking for help.

2. **Eat a healthy diet** - A healthy diet is still important postpartum as it helps you heal and provides nutrients for breastfeeding.

3. **Stay active** - Gentle exercise can help improve mood and aid in recovery.

4. **Seek support** - Postpartum depression is common, so talk to your healthcare provider if you're feeling depressed or anxious.

5. **Practice self-care** - Take time for yourself to do things that make you feel good, whether it's reading a book, taking a bath, or going for a walk.

Real-Life Example: "After giving birth, I made sure to rest and recover and asked for help when I needed it. I also continued to eat a healthy diet and started gentle exercise to aid in my recovery."

21.7.   Conclusion

Pregnancy is an exciting and special time, but it's important to take care of yourself and your baby during this journey. By following a healthy diet, staying active, managing stress, preparing for labor and delivery, and practicing postpartum care, you can have a healthy and happy pregnancy. Remember to talk to your healthcare provider about any concerns or questions you may have, and enjoy this special time in your life.

The End